Drugs And Their Dangers in Papua New Guinea

Philip Kai Morre

A Member of the Simbu Writer's Association.

DEDICATION

For my mama Martha Gambugl.

CONTENTS

ACKNOWLEDGMENTS

My heartfelt gratitude goes to Peter Kepa, Francis Nii and Philip Fitzpatrick for their support in editing and the eventual publication of this book. Without their kind assistance, I don't think this book would have turned out in its current form. Any technical errors are mine.

Prelude

(An awareness campaign).

DEAR young one, student, parent, friend and citizen.

Abuse of drugs and alcohol and their related evils are major issues affecting humanity around the world today and Papua New Guinea is no exception. If you look around the community you live in you will see, smell and breathe drugs every day.

Any foreigners or local visitors coming to the Highlands of PNG for the first time would probably think that the highlanders, mainly the youths, are forever on holiday in paradise enjoying life every day. But the truth is that drugs are causing this temporary merry-go-round mood.

Daily, one can see or smell some form of drug being used or consumed freely and openly in public. You look at one corner or section of the market or public square, you will see youths sitting around smoking, drinking or chewing something that contains or may contain drugs and at most times accompanied by card gambling.

You would see men, women and youths selling bags of *buai*. Among them you would see some elderly people selling bundles of home grown local tobacco commonly known as *brus*. Well, *brus* might contain mild drugs but in the long run it will accumulate and can cause serious bodily damage to the user like cancer.

You look to yet another corner of the public square or market or some other odd spot and you will see empty soft drink plastic containers filled with homebrewed alcohol sold at K5-10 per container. And you would see youths selling marijuana drugs rolled up in cut and sliced pieces of newspapers too.

Some of your dear ones, like your parents, spouse or siblings may have become drug users. Or you may have been the one gotten into the habit of taking drugs.

Well, drugs are good and drugs are bad too. There are good and bad drugs existing in the world. Drugs can be harmful or helpful, depending on how we take them or use them. Most drugs are meant to help us and not to harm or destroy us.

Therefore if we have to use or take drugs, we must do so with caution and advice from experts, we must not overdose ourselves.

This book talks about some of the common drugs we find in the world, both licit and illicit. It discusses the historical uses, the correct purposes, their abuses and the consequences.

It is the writer's hope that after reading this book, people will have learnt something about the different types of drugs and the side effects they cause.

It is also hoped that, although the choice of taking drug or not is an individual's right and freedom to decide, they must not forget that they have a responsibility towards their family, community and the society they belong to and their drug habit should not adversely affect these groups of human beings.

This is the direction of this book and the writer hopes that after one has read, digested and meditated over the information provided, he or she will be placed in a better position to make an informed decision to direct his or her life for the better and not for the worst. The good values of responsibility, discipline, sacrifice, wise thinking, choice making and the basic rights of freedom rests with each and every one.

It is sincerely hoped that the next time the reader thinks of taking a drug, the information contained in this book will remind and caution them to make a sound choice that will be beneficial and not bring destruction to them, their family, the community and society in general.

To our noble and valued off-spring;

son,

    daughter,

        student,

            nephew,

                niece,

                    father,

                        mother,

                            kinsman,

countryman,

    friend

      and stranger foe.

Should you, out of ignorance, unintentionally get yourself hooked up on drugs, homebrew alcoholic beverages or any other form of drugs and you feel that you have become addicted to it and that you have become a slave of it, meaning it controls, drives and forces you around, and you would like to redeem yourself and get out of it and be free again, this information is meant for you to read through and get some helpful ideas.

Do Not Let The Drugs Defeat You For:
You can redeem yourself
You can win over it
You can defeat it
You can change
You can resurrect from it
You were born free
You were meant to be free
You have the right to be free and therefore
You should rightly be free.

Chapter 1

Defining Drugs and Their Functions

A DRUG is any substance that when consumed or taken into the body, alters one or more of the bodily functions. It is a **chemical** that stimulates, depresses or arouses the nervous system or affects the metabolic processes in the human body.

The medicine prescribed by a medical practitioner is a drug, alcohol is a drug, marijuana is a drug, tobacco is a drug, cocaine is a drug, certain mushrooms and plant species are also drugs. Whether they are for good use and socially acceptable or not, all are drugs.

Drugs are grouped into licit and illicit drugs and are classified as safe (beneficial) or unsafe (dangerous) depending on the effects each produces on the human body.

Licit drugs are drugs that are allowed by law to be used or consumed because they are manufactured for good use to benefit people. They are useful and beneficial to human beings.

These drugs are mostly found in the hospitals or health institutions and are also sold in the pharmacy shops. Drugs like alcohol, nicotine and caffeine are included in this category but are different from other substances in terms of socially acceptable drugs.

Illicit drugs are chemicals whose production, consumption and trade are prohibited by law. These are drugs that yield or generate dependency, addiction, tolerance and craving and are made illegal by legislation.

Cannabis, cocaine, morphine, barbiturates, LSD, Amphetamine type stimulants, heroin and hallucinogen drugs are some examples of illicit drugs.

There are numerous types of drugs available. Some drugs are used for relaxation. Some are used for entertainment. Some are used for merriment. Others are used for curing illnesses.

Drugs like coffee and tea contain caffeine while betel nut contains arecoline. While both caffeine and arecoline are alkaloid chemicals (REF); caffeine is a stimulant while arecoline is a psychoactive chemical. Psychoactive agents are also present in pharmaceutical and illicit drugs such as cocaine, heroin, cannabis and lysergic acid diethylamide (LSD). (Handbook for Medical Practitioners, Commonwealth of Australia, 1992, P7).

When drugs are not used properly, like at the right time, in the right amount and for the specific condition it was prescribed for, it becomes overused, abused or wrongly used. The effects experienced by the right use can be rewarding while those suffered by wrong uses can be disastrous or catastrophic.

Many youths and young adults who, in the hope of getting away from small challenges or avoidance of confrontation with the challenges of life, end up taking drugs mildly without knowing or being aware of what it might do to them. They somehow get hooked and many become prisoners of regular or habitual drug taking.

Once the drug user has gotten hooked, their lives are affected and infected and it leads them to a disability of sound reflexes physically, spiritually, mentally and psychologically. It can even create a very strong craving or a drive for taking more drugs and this then leads to **abuse** or **wrong** use.

The word "drug" means medicine. Medicine is found in the hospitals or chemist shops. Medicine is also found in plants.

There are hundreds of drugs known to mankind. Some are traditional medicines made from plants and are taken or used directly.

Some drugs have become commercial commodities like *buai* (betel nut), coffee and tobacco. And other drugs are made in **laboratories** by isolating or extracting them from other chemicals.

A drug store is a chemist or pharmacy shop where one can buy medicine. Different kinds of medicines under different names and labels are sold there. Some medicines are simple and are not dangerous to use, take or consume.

Drugs have certain functions and powers to do something in our bodies when we take them. When we are sick the doctor examines us and prescribes some drugs (prescribed dose) for us to take or use either periodically or daily etc. As long as we follow the prescription or direction of the doctor, the medicine will effectively serve its purpose in our body's systems.

However, if we do not follow the doctor's advice and miss the timing or take less than the prescribed dose etc., the medicine will not work properly and effectively in our body. Consequently our sickness will not get cured. The medicine then becomes wasted or wrongly used or abused.

Depending on the degree and the power of the medicine, it can become legal (legitimate) or illegal (illegitimate).

In recent times the word "drug" has taken on a rather bad meaning and is connected to evil and criminal implication. Even the innocent old grandmother in the house becomes frigid and timid, nervous, frightened and shaky at the hearing of the expression "drug body", "steam body" or *spakman.* These words are used to mean or to describe the kind of attitudes that are usually displayed and shown by **illegal** or **wrong** users of drugs.

Let us give an example of a wrong use of a drug. "Drug body" or "steam body" refers to some people who use or take drugs and medicines, not because they are sick or in need and want of it, but because they want the feelings, the kicks and the elevated self-esteem caused by the drugs. The users get 'nice dreaming work' and are thrilled at the 'imaginations' obtained from the use of the drugs.

The medicine **morphine** is a valuable drug used under strict control by doctors as a painkiller and for therapeutic purposes especially to induce patients to sleep during operations.

When morphine is injected into a patient's body, it sedates and eases the pain. It puts the patient in an unconscious or semi-conscious state depending on the dosage administered. Sometimes it makes people feel good all over. It gives a sort of light headed and dreamy feeling with no problems in life.

While morphine is a good medical drug, some people today take morphine not to remove pain from an operation but only to give themselves these dreamy nice floating feelings.

This is an example of people using medicine, a drug, in a very wrong way. They are abusing the drug or medicine.

Alcohol is meant to be drunk to create merriment to ease the mind and body and to relax. But when people drink a lot of alcohol it affects their brains and other parts of the bodies. This then becomes drug abuse. It is not respecting beer and not using it for the correct purpose.

Marijuana is one of the most dangerous drugs of recent decades. Most young people in Simbu Province and other parts of PNG and Oceania know and use marijuana for many reasons known to them.

Nowadays even elderly people use marijuana to get themselves into the delusive imagination work which makes them feel good all over.

Well, it may be good for the druggies but smoking too much of it can get one hooked. Once you get hooked, it becomes your master and you are its slave. It can have catastrophic and disastrous effects on your brain and body.

The right and freedom to take drug or not and what kind of drug, when and how much to take, rests with us. It is us individuals who decide to destroy or save ourselves. The ability to choose what drugs to take and when and how to take them, to either help or spoil us, is within each of us.

Chapter 2

Why People Use Drugs?

THE main reason for using drugs found everywhere is that people cannot cope with modern life and changes and hence seek an escape mechanism, including taking drugs. Millions of people around the world, including Papua New Guineans, resort to drugs and have created problems for themselves and their families and the society they live in through social, psychological, spiritual, mental and physical disabilities.

A.   Some factors of life that drive people into using or taking of drugs are;

1.   Experimental Use

People try out a drug to experience its effect and decide whether or not to adopt an ongoing pattern of use. Young people use drugs out of curiosity.

2.   Social/Recreational Use

Using drugs as a means of interacting with other people as a sign of friendships, relaxation and enjoyment.

3.   Symptomatic Use

Drugs serve a purpose in reducing unpleasant feelings and provide an escape from problems. Some people use drugs as a medication to cope with life.

4. Dependant Use

A person's body require the drugs to function normally.

5. Peer Pressure

Peer pressure is common among the younger generation. My work mate or school mate or same age group takes the drug so I must take it too is a popular phenomenon.

6. False Belief

Young people take drugs, such as cannabis, with a false hope of curing disease or aiding the brain to find answers to complex questions. Drinking one or two bottles of beer before an exam to reinforce one's thinking capability to pass is one example.

Some youths take drugs to feel older and think big in the adult world.

7. Family Problems

A great number of young people take drugs to cope with family problems, especially marital disputes and divorces.

B. Methods in Which Drugs Enter the Body

There may be other methods where drugs enter the body but the most common ones are:

1. **Oral dose** – through the mouth.
2. **Injection** – direct connection (intravenous) into veins and other parts of the body.
3. **Inhalation** – breathing through the nose into the lungs.
4. **Mucous membranes** – in sites such as the nose, mouth

and rectum. Absorbed through the skin as in nicotine patches.

C. Forms in Which Medicines are Dispensed
(Medical or Pharmaceutical Terms)

Medicines come in different forms in which they are dispensed. The popular forms are;

1. Tablets

These are a solid dosage form in which the medicine is compressed tightly in some sort of medium. Chiloquin, Amoxicillin, Aspirin and many other medicines come in this form.

2. Capsules

These are medicines that are put inside small shells of gelatine, which look like plastic. One end is filled with the medicine and another half is slipped over it. Many antibiotics come in this form.

3. Pills

These are small, round and compressed tablets.

4. Syrups

These are solutions of drugs in a sweet or sugar solution. Many cough medicines come in this way.

Chapter 3

Common Types of Drugs

THERE are many drugs that are considered illegal or unlawful for general use or public consumption because they do harm to the individual user as well as the community and the society through the actions of the addicts. Some examples of the illicit or unlawful drugs are;

1.   Cannabis

Cannabis or marijuana is an herb and is an interesting plant. It contains a highly potent chemical ingredient called **Tetrahydrocannabinol (THC)**.

Cannabis is the most used illicit drug in PNG. A highly potent cannabis propagated through plant breeding techniques is called "**Sinsemilla**" and is widely grown in the highlands.

2.   Cocaine

Cocaine is a white crystal alkaloid powder abstracted from coco leaves. Unlike most other drugs, cocaine can be taken in all the three common processes, namely: inhaling, smoking and intravenous. More on cocaine will be talked about in chapter 6.

3.   Opium

Opium is derived from the seed pod of the opium poppy plant known as *Papaver somniferum*. This drug is not common in PNG.

More on opium will be talked about in chapter 6.

4. Heroin

Heroine is derived from morphine through a chemical process and is much stronger than morphine itself. Although morphine is widely used as a medical drug in PNG, heroine is not so popular.

5. DOM or ST

There are very few legitimate uses of methamphetamine in the medical field. Most of the amphetamines are manufactured in hidden laboratories and go by other street names such as **crystal**. In the Philippines, it is known as "**shabby**."

Dom or **ST** is a type of methamphetamine. It is a hallucinogen drug that can cause serious psychiatric and psychological conditions namely: hallucinations, delusions and paranoia. A person who has consumed it is in the dream world seeing and hearing things that do not exist. This drug has no proper medical use.

6. PCP

PCP is a phencyclidine and is also called "**Angel's Dusk**". It was developed in the 1950s to put people to sleep. When the users wake up they appear delirious or out of their minds.

PCP is easy to make and so by the 1970s it became one of the widely used drugs among users. Today it is mostly used as veterinary medicine to put animals to sleep for operations.

When PCP is taken by a person, he walks like a drunkard. He has disorganized perception and thoughts; drowsiness and an "I could not care less what happens" feeling and attitude.

The heart rate of the person increases and with high doses they can become unconscious and die through depression (suppression) of the respiration.

PCP makes the user insensitive to even very strong pain, hence it can easily be seen why persons with either physical or psychological "pain" would use it.

7.   LSD or D-lysergic Acid Diethylamide

This is a drug that was developed in the 1930s and was not very popular in the medical field. Since 1970 this drug has been banned altogether for use in medicine.

Today it is made in illegal laboratories and comes in the form of a colourless and tasteless liquid or sometimes as white powder.

By adding a drop of sugar or other food the drug can easily be stored on the back of stamps or stickers and therefore is difficult to detect.

People under the influence of LSD will do all sorts of crazy things, such as believing that they can fly and jumping out of the windows of buildings or from the tops of mountains and so on. LSD was very popular to drug addicts at one time.

8.   Methaqualome

This is a hypnotic and legitimate medical drug. However it has now become a drug of abuse. It has obtained its popularity among drug abusers because it is considered an aphrodisiac, meaning it is a sexually stimulating drug.

Users claim that it brings about peaceful relationship with others. But what it actually does is make the user feel and act like a drunk. It causes confusion and disorientation to the mind, thus mentally affecting the user.

9.   Amphetamine

Amphetamine acts as a powerful stimulant which impairs and depresses the Central Nervous System (CNS). At one time they were very popular drugs and were prescribed by doctors to help people reduce their weight. They seemed to give people stronger will power to stay away from eating or abstaining from food.

Because they keep a person alert and awake, students use them to clear their minds before doing their exams or tests. Truck drivers, pilots and night workers use them to keep awake and athletes use them to give them extra strength and energy to perform better in sports.

Amphetamines have limited medical uses and a doctor must exercise care and strict control in administering and monitoring its use in medication.

The ingredients to make amphetamines are easily obtainable and there are many illegal amphetamine factories that turn these drugs out for the black market. It is an addictive and dangerous drug and thus requires control.

The street names of these drugs are Speed, Bennies, Uppers, Co-pilots and Heats.

10. Ecstasy or MDMA

Ecstasy means "a wonderful and delightful time." In English we say a person is in ecstasy meaning he is extremely happy. **MDMA** or **Ecstasy** stimulates the Central Nervous System in a very powerful way.

It was once praised as a medicine that could help people establish good relationships. It was also hailed as an aphrodisiac, which means it was supposed to stimulate people sexually. What it did do was simply put people out of their minds. They couldn't sleep; they were nervous and after the stimulation passed off they were depressed, confused and anxious.

Ecstasy is physically and psychologically addictive.

Chapter 4

Classification of Drugs

THERE are many drugs but the main classifications we will look at are:

1. Stimulant drugs,
2. Narcotic drugs,
3. Hallucinogenic drugs,
4. Designer drugs,
5. Depressive drugs and
6. Seductive drugs.

Everyone, or most people, in the world takes and uses medicine and drugs. A cup of coffee contains a drug. A betel nut contains drugs. A roll of tobacco (*brus*) contains drugs. Cough mixture is made from drugs and a bottle of beer has got drugs in it.

Let us now take a look at what each drug does to the human body.

1. Stimulant Drugs

These are drugs that act to increase body activity. Caffeine in tea and coffee and arecoline in betel nut are classic examples of mild stimulant drugs.

2. Narcotic Drugs (opiates)

An opiate, as a natural or synthetic derivative, when taken in moderate doses dulls the senses and induces consumers to sleep. **Heroin** and **morphine** are examples of this drug.

Their effects may vary, including lack of energy, breathing problems, physical and psychological dependency, craving etc.

Heroin, a derivative of morphine through a chemical process, was discovered in 1874 and is much stronger than morphine itself. It is a narcotic and is produced from morphine while pethidine and methadone are synthetic drugs. (The Drug Offensive, Canberra, Australia, 1984).

Opium is derived from the seed pod of the opium poppy plant. Morphine was isolated from opium at the beginning of 19th Century and got its name after Morpheus, the Greek god of dreams. (The Drug Offensive, Canberra, Australia, 1984).

It is a known fact that drugs produced for therapeutic use or treatment of sick people for relief of pain and other illness are now being abused and there is difficulty in controlling them. As a result these narcotic drugs cause tolerance and dependency.

At a low dose opiates produce euphoria or tranquillity, happiness and a problem-free state of mind. With a higher dose it may produce a good dream and experiences of ecstasy. Then comes drowsiness, dizziness, lack of concentration and disorientation. When overdone it may result in unconsciousness, coma and death. (The Drug Offensive, Canberra, Australia, 1984).

3. Hallucinogen Drugs

These drugs act to change the way the mind works.

Hallucinogenic drugs are sometimes called psychedelic drugs, which in Greek means **mind revealing** because it mainly affects the mind and the brain chemical components. It is a drug that changes the person's perception and causes hallucinations – dreams of seeing and hearing things that do not really exist.

They can change a person's way of thinking, his or her emotions, sense of time and place and can cause abnormal feelings of superiority or heroism. (Issues for Subsistence Abuse, P. 27).

There are many different varieties of hallucinogenic drugs, both natural and manufactured. Natural hallucinogens are found in certain mushrooms, fungi, seeds, leaves of trees, vines and roots.

Other hallucinogens are produced in underground laboratories. (Counselling Issues for Subsistence Abuse, P 27).

Here are some hallucinogen drugs;

➤ **Psilocybin** (magic mushrooms)

Psilocybin is a chemical element found in some bush mushrooms in Central America. In its natural state psilocybin is a white powder and is often sold in dried mushrooms.

Psilocybin belongs to the same group of drugs as LSD and its effects are quite the same. (The Drug Offensive, Canberra, Australia, 1984).

The active ingredient called lysergic acid dimethylamine is found in the Morning Glory plant. (Counselling Issues for Subsistence Abuse, P. 27).

➤ **PCP** (phencyclidine or angel's dusk)

PCP (phencyclidine or angel's dusk) which is derived from the pulp of the peyote cactus is another hallucinogenic drug that can cause hallucinations, i.e. hearing voices that do not exist or seeing colours changing, and aberrations in time and reality. (The Drug Offensive, Canberra, Australia, 1984).

> **LSD**

LSD type psychedelic drugs acting on serotonin cause deep psychological delusionary experiences on the part of the brain, which is crucial for memory and learning.

> **Cannabis**

Cannabis is also known to be a hallucinogenic drug. When a low dose is taken it acts as a depressant drug slowing the bodily functions. When a high dose is taken the consumer goes through day dreaming, experiences delusions, auditory and visual hallucinations and other effects.

> **MDMA** (Methylene Dioxymethamphtamine, ("Ecstasy")

MDMA is an illegal drug manufactured in underground laboratories. It can be taken in tablet, capsule or liquid form.

The effects of **MDMA** vary, depending on the level of dose taken. Lower doses produce a feeling of euphoria. It also causes anxiety, increases heart rate and blood pressure and causes residential head-ache and nausea. (The Drug Offensive, Canberra, Australia, 1984).

Taking more **MDMA,** causes hallucinations which could be visual, auditory or tactile and can lead to other psychological and psychiatric complications.

❖ **Other known hallucinogenic drugs include;**

➢ Dimthyltrypatamin or DMT (Businessman's LSD or businessman's lunch)
➢ Bromo-DMA
➢ Lysergic acid amide - an active ingredient in morning glory plant
➢ Amphetamine – like in low doses, LSD - like in high doses - acting on norepinephrine
➢ Psychedelics
➢ Mescaline (peyote cactus)
➢ DOM or STP (is a synthetic or designer drug product
➢ Myristin and elemican which is an active ingredient in nutmeg similar in structure to mescaline
➢ Psychedelic anaesthetics
➢ Ketamine
➢ General anaesthetics
➢ Atropine (belladonna)
➢ Atropine (natural)
➢ Antihistamines
➢ Other drugs in high doses

4. Designer Drugs/Synthetic Drugs

There are 5 major classes of designer drugs and they are mostly manufactured in underground laboratories. Their names are;

❖ Synthetic Opioids,
❖ Phencyclidine (PCP) Derivatives,
❖ Tryptamines,
❖ Methaqualome Derivatives and
❖ Phenylalkylamines (PAAs).

5. Depressant Drugs
Are drugs that change body activity.

Depressant drugs are substances that decrease the activity of the central nervous system, which affects the bodily functions. Some of these depressant drugs are alcohol, barbiturates and minor tranquilisers.

Alcohol is the most commonly used and is socially acceptable. It is produced by fermentation or distillation of grains, fruits or vegetables.

Alcohol is now produced not only by legitimate government approved liquor breweries but also by illegal home brewers located in the villages.

Barbiturates are depressant drugs derived from barbituric acid. They became popular for medical use but later became a drug of abuse. As a result other safer depressant drugs were produced.

Synthetically produced drugs that are not chemically related to barbiturates are known as non-barbiturate sedatives and include methaqualome, glutethimide and the minor tranquilisers, Valium and Diazepam.

Even though they are medically proven as safe therapeutic drugs, barbiturates have also become abused drugs. (The Drug Offensive, Canberra, Australia, 1984).

Another group of tranquilisers, termed major tranquilisers, are used for the treatment of mental illness. These are strictly controlled by competent medical doctors and applied to their patients under supervision. They should not be confused with minor tranquilisers.

Some of the depressant drugs are controlled by clinics and hospitals and are prescribed as hypnotic or sleeping pills for the relief of anxiety and tension. When abused, depending on the amount of dose (small or moderate), the drugs produce feelings of relaxation and drowsiness. (The Drug Offensive, Canberra, Australia 1984).

6. <u>Sedative Drugs</u>

These drugs act to affect the senses and makes one feel like being in nirvana – at peace and in harmony with the world.

Chapter 5

Drugs Found in Plants

1.   Caffeine

CAFFEINE is a drug most commonly consumed in coffee. Caffeine is a mild stimulant which originates from the seeds of the natural coffee plant. Its botanical name is *Coffea arabilce.*

Caffeine is also found in the leaves of the tea plant, scientifically known as *Thea sinesis* and also in the nuts of the acuminate tree. (Notes, Australia Institute of Counselling in Addiction).

Caffeine is found in concentrated form in coffee, tea, Coca Cola, chocolate and cocoa.

1 cup of coffee = 100-150 mg caffeine.
12 fluid oz. (355 mL) of cola drink = 3-55 mg caffeine.
Chocolate bar = 25 mg caffeine per oz.

➤ Effects of Caffeine

Caffeine stimulates and increases brain and motor activity and alerts and keeps people awake.

➤ Pharmacology and Toxicity

Caffeine is a poison and when intravenously injected it will result in serious health and medical risks. Animals given caffeine in large doses in laboratory experiments resulted in death. It can also be fatal for humans. Some consumers of caffeine-containing substances can build up a tolerance to it.

➢ Psychological Dependence

Caffeine drinkers have reported that they cannot go for long without it. They have to drink in order to get a work started. It keeps their eyes open and mind alert and so forth.

➢ Physiological Dependence

When caffeine is discontinued, withdrawal symptoms develop, especially headaches, stomach pains and mood changes. Also the craving for caffeine or products that contain caffeine is set up.

2. Nicotine

Nicotine is a chemical ingredient in tobacco plants that are grown in every part of the world, including PNG and is classified as a legalised drug in terms of social acceptability.

In PNG many people cultivate tobacco and the leaves are dried in fire places or by the heat of the sun. When the leaves are thoroughly dry they are sold at the local markets, either in bundles of leaves or rolled up in newspaper.

When tobacco is processed as cigarettes in a factory it is treated with other chemicals, thus increasing the risk of cancer.

Nicotine is a poisonous chemical that causes severe bodily harm, especially in stimulating the nervous system, increasing the heart rate, raising blood pressure and dilating the blood vessels under the skin that can cause wrinkles.

Nicotine causes addiction like many other drugs and the

withdrawal symptoms are quite severe. It is life threatening because it causes diseases like cancer and emphysema. Treating smoking related illnesses costs the community greatly.

Tar from tobacco smoking is a black sticky chemical substance that damages the throat, affects the tissues in the lungs and causes breathing problems. Tar is also a cancer causing substance in smokers. (Health Promotion Services, Health Department of Western Australia, 1997).

3. <u>Other Drugs found in Plants</u>

➤ Marijuana

Marijuana is the name referred to the dry leaves and flowers of the cannabis plant that are smoked. The name marijuana is derived from the Spanish phrase for **"Mary-Jane"**. This drug is discussed in more detail in chapter 6.

➤ Cocaine

Cocaine is a white crystal alkaloid powder extracted from the leaves of the coco plant. This drug is discussed in more detail in chapter 7.

➤ Opium

Opium is a narcotic drug. The term narcotic originates from the Greek word **narcosis,** which means put to sleep.

Drugs or chemicals like heroin, morphine, codeine and other seductive pills are derivatives of opium. Opium is discussed in more detail in chapter 7.

Chapter 6

The Drug Cannabis

1   <u>Discovery and Its Use</u>

BELOW are the three common species of cannabis.

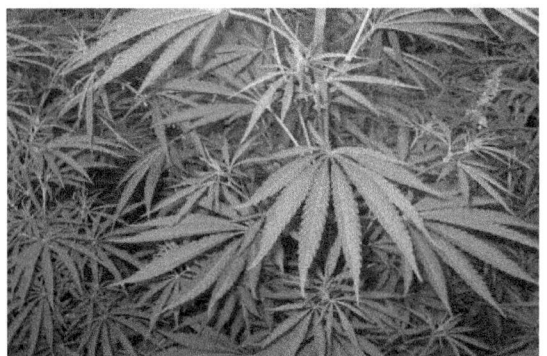

Figure 1: This is Cannabis sativa.

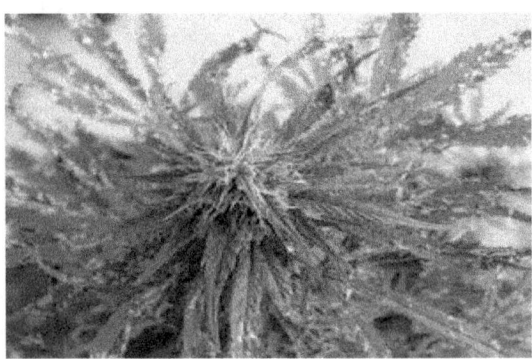

Figure 2: This is Cannabis indica.

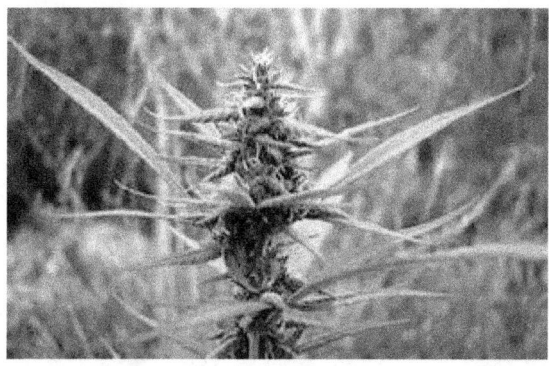

Figure 3: This is Cannabis ruderalis.

Cannabis is believed to be originated from Central Asia, dating back to the 5th Century BC.

Chinese doctors in the ancient times used cannabis as an anaesthetic or painkiller to relieve pain during surgery. The plant was known to contain pharmacological chemical properties for therapeutic use or treatment of patients at that time.

In the Middle East cannabis plants are used to manufacture twine ropes or fibre. It has many uses and is considered as a good plant. (Cannabinaceae, Backer, Heematede P: 221-222, December 1965).

The Scythians in the fifth century BC used cannabis for religious and cultural activities, like burials and rituals as well as using the leaves for steam bathing. (Monograph 98 on the Hidden Population, 1990).

In India, the Hindu monks used cannabis to overcome hunger and thirst while meditating and fasting. They thought that cannabis was a miracle or wonder drug and a gift from God to use it for many purposes. (The Drug Offensive, 1987).

In the contemporary world, cannabis has lost its therapeutic values and is not considered a good pharmaceutical drug any longer. Research and studies have revealed that the cannabis plant grown today is more psychoactive potent and is much more dangerous. It damages the brain chemistry and other parts of the body.

Plant breeding techniques has increased chemical potency of plants causing greater destruction of human health and lives. (Gabriel Nahas, 1990).

The famous Swedish botanist, Carl Linus, first discovered the cannabis plant and named it *Cannabis sativa*, derived from the Spanish word **Canavere**. (Line, 1753).

Later on another famous French botanist, Jean Lamark, discovered another species and named it *Cannabis indica* after India where he first lived and discovered the plant. (Lamark, 1783).

An unknown Russian botanist discovered another species and named it *Cannabis ruderalis*. There could be more species. Botanical research and studies are still going on.

Up until now these three main species of cannabis are grown in many parts of the world especially in the temperate zones of South American countries, including Colombia, Peru, Guatemala, Argentina, Brazil, Mexico, Bolivia and Jamaica, and also in the South East Asian countries like Cambodia, Lao, Myanmar, Malaysia, Philippines, Indonesia, East Timor, Vietnam and Thailand. South Pacific countries, including Papua New Guinea, also cultivate and produce high quality cannabis.

Through genetic plant breeding the underground scientists have developed a hybrid cannabis called *sinsemilla*, which means "**without seeds**". This hybrid cannabis, which is also grown in

PNG, mostly in the highlands, especially Simbu and the Eastern Highlands and Western Higlands provinces where the climate is temperate, has high psychoactive or psychedelic ingredients and chemical potency.

The **Tetrahydrocannabinol** (Delta 9) or THC percentage in *sinsemilla* is between 20 to 30 percent, which is very high. (UNCP Report 2002).

The THC content (chemical ingredient) of cannabis grown in PNG is highly risky. (UNCP Report,1992, P.42).

There are probably other chemical contents which have been increased but they are not yet known.

The nickname given to the plant by the hidden populations of the drug sub-culture, namely drug addicts, drug dealers and cultivators is New Guinea Gold. (Notes, J Denials, Lae Drug Conference, (1990).

One of the botanists or plant specialists who did extensive research on cannabis in the highlands of Papua New Guinea, E.E. Henty, discovered that the most popular cannabis plant species grown in the highlands of PNG is *Cannabis sativa*. (Cannabis in PNG, Benjamin Thomas).

The other species of cannabis are not yet established or remain isolated.

There are many street names for cannabis known among the hidden population in the drug culture. Pot, bong grass, joint, Bomai *brus*, Maria, Mary-Jane and butt are some of these names.

2   Pharmaceutical (Chemical Properties in Cannabis)

Cannabis is the scientific name given to this herb plant.

Marijuana is the name of the dry leaves of cannabis that is smoked. When using marijuana, the users' problems and worries appear to magically disappear and they feel like as if they are on top of the world.

There are more than 400 chemicals found in the cannabis plant and most of these are remote and isolated. Of all these, there are 60 cannabinoids but only 16 main ones have been isolated in laboratories.

It is not known whether any of these cannabinoids isolated by scientists contain therapeutic chemicals or drugs for treating patients. (British Journal of Psychiatry, P 41).

The main cannabinoid that is an active ingredient is called "tetrahydrocannabinol (THC)" or colloquially Delta 9. THC is the psychoactive ingredient found in cannabis. (Handbook for Medical Practitioners, Commonwealth of Australia, 1992).

The quality and potency of the drug depends on how and where the plant is grown and how well it is prepared.

The highlands region of PNG, where the climate is temperate and the general condition of the soil is good, the hybrid *sinsemilla* cannabis grows very well. It is an easily adaptable plant and does not require insecticide or fertilizer.

Researchers point out that cannabis remains a plant of its own and can be classified under stimulant, depressant or hallucinogen.

Because cannabis is changing its characteristics in the

revolutionary process we are now experiencing more and more new problems associated with it. This includes its increased chemical potency due to scientific engineering such as cloning and new methods of preparation. (UNIDCP Report, 1992, P 420).

3   How Marijuana is Prepared and Taken

❖ **Marijuana**

Marijuana can be smoked using the dried leaves, flowering tips, seeds and stems of the cannabis plant. It is rolled and smoked in newspaper or smoking pipes, which are the most common ways among users, especially the young people.

❖ **Hashish**

Hashish is the name given to concentrated type of cannabis made by compressing cannabis resins from the flowering tops into small blocks and eaten as biscuits. Hashish is much more powerful than marijuana, containing 5 to 10 times more potent THC. (The Drug Offensive, 1987).

❖ **Hashish Oil**

Hashish oil is obtained by compressing cannabis into a chemical solvent and evaporating the solvent to obtain an oil concentrate.

❖ **The Crude and Blunt**

The terms **crude** or **blunt** refer to the increased potency of new marijuana smoking forms. They include removing the manufactured tobacco content in a cigarette and refilling the paper with a potent marijuana mixed with chopped dry tobacco leaf. Very high effects are produced by this method.

Consumers also report that 'pillie blunts', using cigars are an effective way of taking the drug. (The Addiction Letter, Vol. 9, No. 11, November, 1993).

There are other means of increasing potency and new methods are being invented every year as scientific knowledge and ideas increase. Of one such invention is the bucket bombing (water pipe) method which is popular in the Simbu and the Eastern Highlands provinces.

Individual users invent new methods of using cannabis mainly to increase the potency to feel the maximum effect. Some users boil cannabis plants like tea or coffee, and add sugar and mix it with alcoholic drinks. A young woman died of an overdose by boiling alcohol with cannabis plants in the remote village of Koge in 1991. (Phillip K. Morre, Times of PNG, 1992).

The injury risk associating with this method is very high. Those who use it normally experience psychosis, unconsciousness, hallucinations, shock, coma and other medical and psychiatric complications. Several people, especially youths between the age of 12 and 16 years, have died of extreme shock. (The Addiction Letter, Vol. 9, No. 11, November 1993).

4   The Effects of Marijuana

Marijuana, like any other mood-altering drug, deranges the levels of neuron transmitters in the brain cells. The neurotransmitters then malfunction or do not operate as they should in the brain chemistry system.

The black tar THC deposited in the spaces between the brain cells of marijuana users stay there for many days. The THC deposits in the brain cells disrupt the natural flow of the neuron transmitters or chemical messages to all parts of the body. (British Journal of

Psychiatry, 1993, p 141).

THC is the mind-altering, fat soluble ingredient in cannabis, which stays for a long time in the brain cells, reproductive system (testes and ovaries), lungs, nerves and other parts of the body.

Once THC gets into the cells it cannot get back into the blood stream like other drugs do.

Alcohol, for example, leaves the body quickly because it is soluble in the blood stream.

Because marijuana is a fat-soluble drug it circulates, burns and leaves the body slowly. Marijuana can be detected in the blood or in a urine sample 21 to 28 days after it is used. (Huw Thomas, British Journal of Psychiatry, 1993).

Smoking Marijuana increases the heart rate and blood pressure. It has cardiovascular effects. Smoking more means the effects will be greater and last longer.

Marijuana will cause the heart beat to increase to 30 beats per minute and sometimes 50 beats per minute and continues for a long period of time, causing bodily damage. (Hand book for Medical Practitioners, 1993, P 59).

Marijuana also affects the reproductive system of both men and women users. Men who have used marijuana have been shown to have low sperm counts and lower testosterone levels. Part of the male hormones essential for sex determination or conception is destroyed. (Handbook for Medical Practitioners, 1993, P. 53-54).

THC reduces the level of hormones in the female reproductive system. They may also experience irregular menstrual cycles.

Smoking marijuana is very risky to the unborn child as it affects the hormones that are essential for the normal growth of the fertilized egg in the uterus.

THC can also reduce the production of hormones in marijuana users and in the foetuses of pregnant users.

The THC in the mother's blood is carried to the blood of the unborn. The mother can give birth to babies with deformities (loss of weight, small heads etc.), just like what happens in those babies born of alcoholic mothers with fatal alcoholic syndrome. (Handbook for Medical Practitioners, 1993, P 53-54).

It is very risky for people with psychological problems, people prone to risk taking and those seeking escape from reality to take marijuana.

They become more irresponsible and put themselves at a high risk of injury. They are likely to experience deep psychological and psychiatric disturbances. Severe cases of psychosis, manic depression, paranoia, delirium tremens and hallucinations have been reported in people using marijuana under such conditions. (British Journal of Psychiatry, 1993. P 41).

Some smokers have reported that smoking marijuana helps them to recall memories of past experiences and even makes their minds clearer. There is no scientific evidences to date to verify such claims.

In reality, most smokers' long term memory is adversely affected. They cannot recall or remember events, time, places, people's names and other things.

Some cannabis smokers experience heightened perceptions, such as seeing colours more brightly, or altered perceptions, such as seeing objects looking out of shape and size that keep moving and tricking the eyes.

At high dose, people have experienced visual, auditory and tactile hallucinations meaning seeing, hearing and feeling things that do not exist. (British Journal of Psychiatry, 1993, P 648-9).

Researches and studies by various experts have shown that marijuana impairs both long and short term memory because THC stays longer in the brain cells – up to 5-6 weeks even with a single dose. THC is deposited in the spaces between the brain cells and limbic system disrupting the natural flow of chemical messages or neurotransmitters. (Microsoft Encarta Encyclopaedia, Oxford Scientific Films/Landon).

The hippocampus is another component of the brain limbic system that is crucial for learning, memorising and the integration of sensory experiences with emotions and motivations. Marijuana induces euphoria (a false feeling of good) with toxic effects of THC on the brain nerve cells. (National Institute on Drug Abuse, Rockville, Maryland, 1989).

There is a theory that cannabis consumption leads to schizophrenia, (split personality) or a serious kind of mental problem or psychosis resembling schizophrenia. It has been reported that those who have been affected may have a predisposition towards psychological and psychiatric problems or behaviours and vice versa.

Also there is an increase in suicide after the consumption of cannabis. According to experts cannabis is the drug that affects the brain much more than any other parts of the body. (Dr.

Gabriel Nahas, Queensland Health Department Report, 1991).

❖ The Lung

Researchers at the University of California have indicated that smoking 1 to 2 joints of marijuana daily will have the same cancer risk as smoking 5 cigarettes a day. THC and other chemicals in cannabis especially the 'tar' affect the lungs. This black substance which is 10 times more potent than cigarettes can cause cancer, bronchitis, emphysema and other medical complications. (National Institute on Drug Abuse, Rockville, Maryland, 1989).

❖ The Heart

Smoking cannabis increases the heartbeat by as much as 50 percent especially with high dose. Chest pain is also reported in some users who may have poor blood supply to the heart.

Heart is an important organ in the body that supports life and when chemicals disturb its normal function, life is destroyed.

❖ The Immune System

It is a known fact that THC penetrates the immune system weakening its power to fight against all sorts of sicknesses in the human body including HIV/AIDS virus. Chemicals in cannabis especially THC is an immune weakening substance. It penetrates and interferes with the body's immune's response to various infections and diseases. The possibility of the cannabis consumers contacting HIV/AIDS is high because of risky sexual behaviour such as unprotected sex.

❖ The Reproductive System

In men, constant use of marijuana can lead to reduction of

testosterone level, produce low sperm count and malformation or defective sperm not healthy for fertilization in women.

THC also reduces the erection capacity or causes impotence problems and pre-mature ejaculations during sexual intercourse.

In women, THC disrupts the natural flow of menstrual cycles. THC also travels through the placenta and causes deformities in the unborn similar to foetal alcohol syndrome.

The luteinizing hormone which is important for implantation of the fertilized egg in the uterus is affected when smoking marijuana. A single dose of marijuana during the lacteal phase of menstrual cycle suppressed the level of the hormone affecting the reproductive system in women. There are also higher rates of spontaneous abortions, foetal deaths and still births (FAS) (Handbook for Medical Practitioner, 1993, P 53-54).

Chapter 7

The Drug Cocaine

1   What is Cocaine?

COCAINE is a white crystal alkaloid powder extracted from coco leaves. It is called *enychioxylon cola* (cocaine hydrochloride). (Video Encyclopaedia on psychoactive drugs).

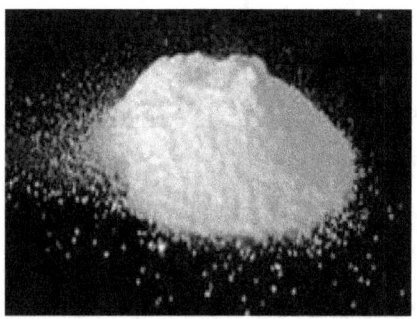

Figure 4: White crystal alkaloid Cocaine powder.

The discovery and origin and its historical use date back to 3000 BC or more when the Incas (South American Indians) used cocaine for ceremonial and religious rituals.

In 1504, a Spanish ethno-botanist by the name of Amerigo Vespucci gave an account or testimony of what red Indians on an island in South America would normally do. They would put coca leaves and powdered lime into their mouth and chew it like betel nut (*buai*) almost every day.

When he asked for drinking water they gave him lime and coca leaves instead and Vespucci guessed or worked out that they kept these in their mouths to alleviate their thirst. (Research Monograph 98 on the Hidden Population, 1990, P 15).

The Red Indians considered cocaine as a gift from God.

In 15-1600 AD the Spanish explorers and settlers realized that the Indians would never work in the mines without taking coca. So they allowed them to chew or gave the Indians coca leaves as part of their wages.

When asked, the Indians would reply that chewing coca leaves prevented them from getting thirsty and hungry and gave them more strength and energy to work in the mines or do other manual work. (Monograph 98 on the Hidden Population, 1990, P 15).

Albert Numen was one of the first German scientists to purify cocaine and isolate some of its chemicals and pharmaceutical properties.

The famous Austrian neurologist, psychiatrist and founder of psychoanalytic theory, Sigmund Freud, published a paper called "Ueber Coca" in 1884. In his paper, Sigmund stressed the need to use cocaine for therapeutic use and called it a "wonder drug" or "miracle drug". He used it to treat patients who were on psychotherapy or had neurotic disorders, including depression and fatigue. (Video Encyclopaedia on psychoactive drugs).

Sigmund Freud also used cocaine himself and recommended it to his friends and patients. One of his friends Dr. Ernst Von Fleischi Marxow almost died from an overdose because of the lack of knowledge about its side effects.

It was then realized that cocaine was, in fact, a dangerous drug that could cause bodily damage and other side effects. (Video Encyclopaedia on psychoactive drugs).

Sigmund's research and writings encouraged a lot of scientists and doctors in Europe and Germany. One of them was Albert Numen, a German doctor who used cocaine as an anaesthetic or pain killer and as treatment of eye diseases and other medical problems. Cocaine became widely used for the treatment of patients at that time and was thought to have a powerful therapeutic use. (Video Encyclopaedia on psychoactive drugs).

In 1886 cocaine was used in cola drinks like Coca Cola and as a "tonic for people who were easily tired". Cola was also used for people with headaches, hysteria and melancholic.

In 1903 Coco-Cola replaced cocaine with caffeine. It was also called an "Intellectual Drink" and used among people of high status and intellectuals in Europe and elsewhere. (Video encyclopaedia on psychoactive drugs).

Cocaine acts as both a stimulant and depressant of the central nervous system (CNS) and also acts as anaesthetic making people sleepy and weak.

The three common methods of using cocaine are inhaling, smoking and injecting. Whether it is smoked, injected or inhaled, the effects are quite the same. (Video Encyclopaedia on Psychoactive drugs).

❖ Crack or Freebase Cocaine

Crack or rock is another form of cocaine normally referred to as "freebase cocaine". It is different in the way it is prepared and much more potent than other types of cocaine.

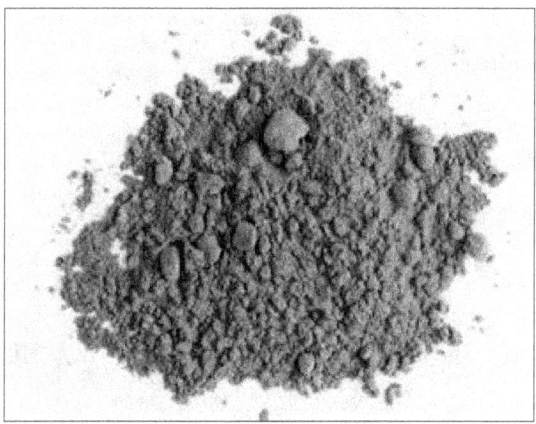

Figure 5: This is also cocaine but in rock or earth form commonly known as rock.

Cocaine is mixed with a solution of baking soda or ammonia in water and is heated. After the water dries up a hard paste remains. This hard paste is then cut into chips or rocks that resembles small chunks of gravel.

The chunks are smoked in water pipes or in cigarettes and are much more dangerous because the drug reaches the brain chemistry system within seconds and produces euphoria (feeling good) which can last for 3 to 5 minutes. (USA Department of Education, 1987).

Crack cocaine is highly addictive and the craving for it is powerful and life threatening to users. Crack users become paranoid and their minds are filled with false beliefs of hope and enjoyment of life.

It also contains powerful addictive properties that normally pushes the users to take more and more crack, putting themselves at high risk of injury. Because of the hankering, the crack users are forced to beg or steal from others in order to buy the drug to support their cravings and consequently their socio-economic wellbeing dwindles. (USA Department of Education, 1987).

2   How Cocaine is Used

There are three methods of using cocaine hydrochloride;

1.   By Sniffing

The fumes or powder form of cocaine is sniffed into the nostrils and with this method the effects are very fast; it appears within seconds. The feeling of euphoria is followed by depression and other psychological and medical effects.

2.   By Swallowing

Cocaine is also used in tablet form and capsules. It is used like taking a tablet or capsule when one is sick. It takes minutes for the effects to come on.

3.   By Injecting

Cocaine is also injected intravenously into the veins. This is the most risky method because sharing the needles with someone who is HIV positive will spread the virus. It has been medically proven that HIV/AIDS is often spread through contaminated needles.

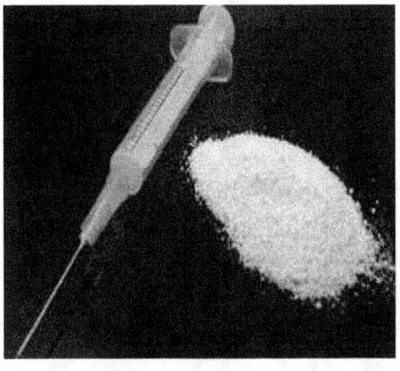 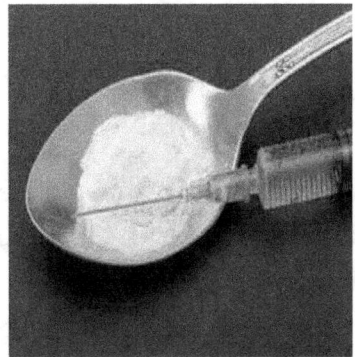

Figures 6 & 7: These pictures show intravenous drug use via injection.

3   The Effects of Cocaine

The effects of cocaine vary from person to person depending on;

➢ The amount of cocaine taken by a person.

➢ The method of how the cocaine is prepared and taken.

➢ The person's physical build, size, weight and health conditions.

➢ The person's mood swings, psychological or personality type or mind set.

➢ The length of time that the person has been taking the drug.

➢ Poly abuse, like taking cocaine with other drugs like marijuana.

➢ The physical and social environmental influence.

Cocaine is a stimulant drug that acts on the central nervous system (CNS) and it also acts as an anaesthetic (pain killer) that numbs the bodily tissues.

When it is injected, inhaled or smoked, the immediate effects are euphoria, feeling good or ecstatic, an increase of energy, alertness and a feeling of confidence.

It also increases sexual desire and appetite and causes visual, tactile and auditory hallucinations and delusions. Hallucinations mean seeing, hearing, smelling and feeling things that do not exist or are unreal. Hallucinations are a mental disorder that are caused by taking drugs. (National Clearing for Alcohol and Drug information, Rockville, USA).

The effects of euphoria or feeling good fades away quickly or suddenly, depending on how the cocaine was taken.

It takes only 10 seconds or less for the effects of cocaine to come on after taking it, hence it is the most preferred drug for inhaling.

When injecting it takes 20 seconds to penetrate the brain chemistry system disrupting the flow of neurons via the neuron transmitters responsible for chemical and electrical messages within the brain and other parts of the body.

Snorting is another common way of taking cocaine and it takes 3 minutes to feel the effects. (National Clearing for Alcohol and Drug Information, Rockville, USA).

The occasional use of cocaine produces nasal congestion and a runny nose. A possible consequence of chronic cocaine snorting is ulceration of the mucous membrane of the nose.

Heavy cocaine snorting can cause the nasal septum to permanently collapse.

Higher doses of cocaine can have toxic effects. People can die of an overdose as a result of respiratory and or cardiac arrest.

(National Clearing for Alcohol and Drug Information, Rockville, USA).

Cocaine can create physical and psychological dependence and when quitting the user will go through severe withdrawal symptoms because it is a powerful and psychologically addictive drug.

When cocaine concentrates directly on the dopamine in the pleasure centre in the brain, it stimulates and produces a well-being or euphoria feeling. It creates 'feeling really good and ecstatic' all over.

This feeling good is like a hook that forces the user to develop intense cravings or desire to get more and more cocaine to feel the same effect. More cocaine becomes necessary to generate the same level of pleasure, which can lead into physical and psychological dependency or addiction. (National Clearing for Alcohol and Drug Information, Rockville, USA).

Addiction to cocaine or crack is very painful and a nightmare for the users. The very moment one uses cocaine, there is no way to stop or escape from this monster. It is the devil you know, that will remain in you as long as you are hooked giving you all the problems in the world you can think of.

At first, a false feeling of euphoria (feeling good) is set up and you feel really great (Hero). You feel that you are somebody special and at peace with the world.

Then severe depression and craving follows with a compulsive desire to take more and more cocaine to feel the same effect. (National Clearance for Alcohol and Drug Information, Rockville, USA).

Then within minutes, after the effects are gone, you feel really down and depressed again so you need more cocaine to feel good again. Craving for more cocaine becomes a real burden and nightmare.

Your body cries out for more and more doses of cocaine or crack that stimulates you to feel the same glorious feeling that you experienced earlier.

Cocaine crack is also called an 'upper and downer'. It makes you feel good when you are high and when you are down it make you feel more terrible and really bad. You feel the urge and strong desire to take more and more within a short period of time to support your craving, increased tolerance, dependency and addiction. (National Clearing for Alcohol and Drug Information, Rockville, USA).

4   Tolerance and Dependence

The cocaine addict develops tolerance, meaning that they need more and more cocaine to feel the same high effects. And each time they take cocaine, the dose required to achieve the same level of effects goes higher. The user's physical, emotional and social lives become dictated by the drug.

The more they use cocaine the more they will find it difficult to stop because their body, mind and thoughts are constantly focussed on it. The cocaine addict becomes a slave to this non-living material like a slave master forcing him to face lots of problems until he or she is dead. (National Clearing for Alcohol and Drug Information, Rockville, USA).

The **Compulsive Craving,** or strong desire to take more and more cocaine, has cost the health and lives of many people and has left them in great financial debt. Crack addicts enter a kind of deadly circle and their lives are thrown away into hell and they become slaves to their addiction.

Slaves have no freedom to make choices or escape from experiencing hardship and danger. The cocaine or crack addict gives up his or her morals, knowledge, rationality, wealth, experiences, personality and spirituality. Most of all, being a human being comprised of a body, spirit and soul created in the image of God is completely destroyed and devalued.(National Clearing for Alcohol and Drug Information Rockville, USA).

The craving for more drugs punishes or pushes the addicted user to an extreme where he or she no longer exists as a human person created in the image of God. His or her dignity as a human person and his values as a free moral and spiritual being no longer exists.

Instead he or she is dragged into serfdom with no strength left to free himself or herself from this monster. (National Clearing for Alcohol and Drug Information, Rockville, USA).

Crack cocaine sets up a **vicious cycle** when it aggravates the biochemical system in the brain rather than relieving it. It pushes the user to take more and more until the drug supplies are run out and all the money is gone. The user then suffers extreme depression, paranoia, delusive distortions, tremors and other psychiatric and psychological problems. It even leads the user to unconsciousness, coma and death.

The drug pusher, on the other hand, gets rich (National Clearing for Alcohol and Drug Information, Rockville, USA).

The **withdrawal symptoms** appear when the drug is discontinued or reduced in dose. The users experience continuous nightmares and symptoms like depression, anxiety, weakness (tiredness), feeling sick, body and head aches, sleeping disorders (sleepless nights), facing and having day dreaming experiences and the craving for the drug. (National Clearing for Alcohol and Drug Information, Rockville, USA).

Chapter 8

More Information on Crack Cocaine

1   The Physical Effects

A crack user suffers from physical effects ranging from lung damage to high blood pressure, tremors and compulsions. It can bring physical injuries, coma and death. Crack can cause suffocation and brain seizures and a lot of young people are sent to their graves for excessive use or overdosing on crack.

❖ **The Overdose**

Users can go through toxic effects because of the concentrated vapour that enters the bloodstream and the brain. Many young people die of crack cocaine overdoses.

❖ **Heart Attack**

Crack cocaine use can over burden the heart and can be fatal for both young and old users.

❖ **Stroke**

Crack cocaine can cause high blood pressure and bursting of the blood vessels in the brain. The crack user can be physically paralysed or die from stroke. This can apply to any person with just one high dose.

❖ Pregnancy

Cocaine use affects the mother and the unborn child. Studies have shown that cocaine use during pregnancy causes miscarriages, premature deliveries, deformities and other complications. Babies born of mothers who use cocaine and are cocaine addicts are under weight and will face behavioural problems.

2   <u>The Psychological Effects</u>

Crack cocaine is a drug that disturbs the brain and affects the user severely, causing delirium tremens, hallucinations and seeing and hearing voices that do not exist. It also causes anxiety, sleeping problems and memory loss and etc.

Crack cocaine users exhibit violent behaviour and deviant personalities. They cannot tell the difference between right and wrong, good and bad and harmful and not harmful etc. Some users experience extreme depression. They worry and live in fear and feel like committing self-injury or suicide. (US Department of Education).

Crack cocaine looks harmless and the habit is cheap at the beginning, costing only a few kina, but most users don't know that this white, small crystalline substance is cunning and potently dangerous enough to punish the user and make them become the most foolish man or woman with no dignity at all.

While it costs less in the beginning, once the user is hooked on the habit and regularly consumes it, it will cost more and more money beyond his or her means. The user will even become a beggar, asking people in a forceful way for money and even stealing to buy more crack drugs. (US Department of Education).

Crack cocaine spoils the brain biochemistry system and sets up a false hope of feeling good and then develops a craving for more and more. Most crack users feel the urge to take in more and more and it develops into a vicious cycle.

Crack cocaine disturbs the natural functions of the biochemical system to the brain so that more of the drug adds more craving rather than relieving it. (US Department of Education)

3   Signs of Crack or Cocaine Use

You can easily observe the changes in physical appearance, changes in personality and changes in behaviour of a crack user.

Crack users show no interest in their work and are often restless and lazy. They feel depressed and feel isolated from the rest of the community.

They are violent and aggressive towards their own families and friends. They often show no interest in doing good things but are often involved in antisocial behaviour.

For students who consume cocaine, they are absent from classes, their marks drop and they show no interest in learning and fall asleep in class. (US Department of Education).

Chapter 9

The Drug Opium and Its Derivatives

AS noted earlier, opium is called **opium poppy** and its scientific name is *Papaver sominiferum*. Opium poppy is a narcotic drug originating from the Greek word **narcosis,** which means put to sleep.

Opium poppy and derivatives refers to opium and other chemicals both illicit and licit that are isolated or extracted from opium poppies, including drugs like heroin, morphine, codeine and other seductive pills.

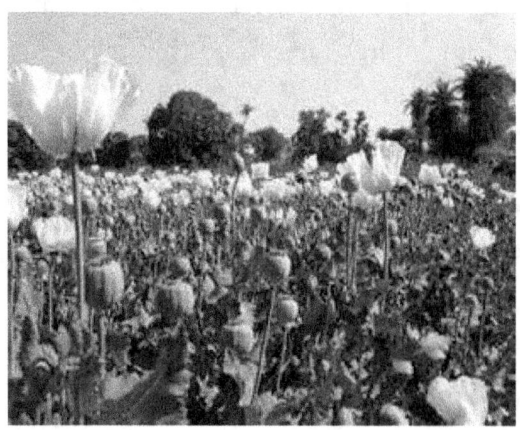

Figure 8: This is the poppy plant the drug opium is derived from.

Opium poppy plants were discovered and used in the Middle East and South East Asia some 3,000 years ago. Chinese monks in the ancient times used opium poppies for religious and ritual purposes.

Opium is the liquid or juice that is pressed out from the poppy plant and was used as a pain killer by ancient Greek doctors when operating on patients. Paracelsus, a Swiss German Renaissance physician, botanist, alchemist, astrologer, and general occultist, who founded the discipline of toxicology introduced opium in Europe for therapeutic use around 1525/30.

Sertuner, a German scientist in 1803 isolated a chemical from the opium plant and called it **morphine,** meaning 'dreams' in Greek after Morpheus, the Greek god of dreams. Later other chemicals were derived from morphine in laboratories for therapeutic use, including **codeine,** which was discovered 1848 and used in cough medicine.

Despite being used as a treatment for various illnesses, opium was known to cause addiction. The Chinese emperors recognised that opium was a dangerous drug that caused a lot of physical, medical and social problems and imposed laws to control it. The laws imposed penalties on both the consumers as well as the cultivators.

Britain went to war with China twice over the issue of opium production. These were called the **opium wars,** with the first from 1839 to 1842 and the second from 1856 to 1858. China had stopped opium production for trade with India and England and many British trading companies lost money. After the wars, despite being won by Britain, the opium trade never picked up again due to the fact that people had recognised the many psycho-social and medical problems associated with the drug. A popular revolt by the people forced the government to immediately stop opium production in 1870.

In 1874, an English scientist, C. Wright, boiled morphine with another chemical called **acetic acid** and produced white crystals called **di-a-ctyl-morphine.** His dog fell unconscious and died after being experimented on with the drug and he did not continue his research work because of the side effects.

A German pharmaceutical company did further research and produced the drug called **di-acetyl-morphine heroin** and described it a wonderful anaesthetic or pain killing drug.

The side effects of using this drug become real for many users. Many became highly addicted with no treatment and cure available. The government intervened with regulations and laws that forbade the production and using of the drug. As a result the company stopped production of the drug completely.

Today Afghanistan and Myanmar are the main producers of illegal opium for underground international marketing and consumption. The term 'golden crescent' (meaning half moon shape) refers to countries or geographical locations, including Afghanistan, Pakistan, Iraq, Iran and Turkey that produce opium.

However, most of the opium production comes from Afghanistan with almost 70 percent due to 3 main structural and underlining problems. (Global Illicit Drug Trends, 2001).

➢ The government is too weak to control its population and the drug problems.

➢ Poverty is the main factor that allows people to grow opium as a cash crop for marketing.

➢ Constant political and civil arrest in the area has displaced the people and they do not have farming land readily available for sustainable agriculture farming so they resort to opium cultivation for quick profits.

The structural problem in Afghanistan is a very complex issue that needs more time and resources to analyse, especially the economic, social, political, agricultural, land, infrastructure and geographical factors that lead to opium cultivation. International assistance is required to solve and reduce the demand and supply. (Global Illicit Drug Trends, 2001).

The next largest producer of opium is Myanmar. Myanmar was influenced by Chinese traders, the first cultivators of opium for trade with other countries.

People in the isolated mountain regions of Myanmar also use opium for religious and rituals purposes. Myanmar has experienced a lot of problems with illegal opium production associated with HIV AIDS and crime.

It is now a real international concern where trafficking of opium and other hard drugs, like Amphetamine Type Stimulants (ATS), are smuggled via South East Asia to Indonesia and the Papua New Guinea border and to the Torres Strait Islands. Due to the lack of proper surveillance systems, security measures, man power and logistics problems, international drug traders and syndicates regard PNG as an ideal transit point to Australia and New Zealand and other countries of the pacific. (Global Illicit Drug Trends, 2011).

Chapter 10

The Amphetamine Type Stimulants (ATS)

ATS in tablet form.

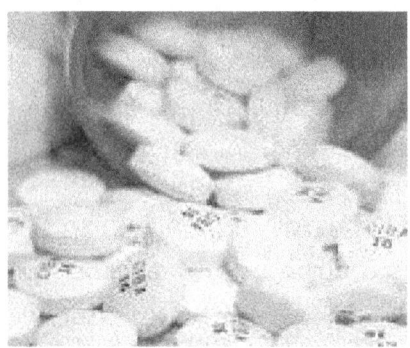 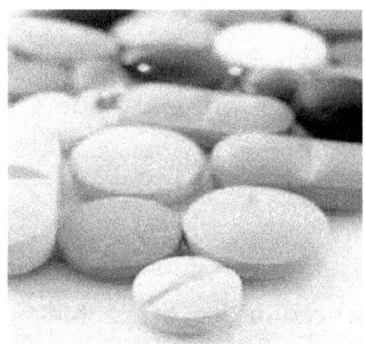

Figure 9 & 10: These photos show the drug amphetamine tablets.

THE Amphetamine Type Stimulant (ATS) is a synthetic drug of recent decades that is manufactured in underground laboratories, mostly in South East Asia.

ATS and other synthetic drugs are falsely conceived as less harmful than other drugs because they are mostly in tablet form, which can be swallowed rather than injecting or smoking.

While the users might have false hopes of feeling good, enjoying themselves and feeling confident and energetic, dependency develops very fast bringing serious mental health problems, severe brain damage, paranoia, kidney failure, internal bleeding and other medical complications. (UN office of Drugs and Crime, November, 2003).

The use of ATS and its production and trafficking are complicated and beyond our scope of knowledge to date. To fully understand the nature of these drugs is difficult and the law enforcing bodies cannot do much to stop the trafficking or the underground ATS manufacturing laboratories.

ATS is now seen as an epidemic that affects millions of people. It is especially spreading very fast among the young generations across the Asian countries, America, Europe and other parts of the world that have experienced discontinued cultural and moral values and peer pressure. (UN Office of Drugs and Crime, November, 2003).

These synthetic drugs can also be easily modified so new forms, such as high **purity crystalline methamphetamine,** developed and mostly found in South East Asian countries.

There is also an added and new burden in the form of another synthetic drug called **crystal meth.** This is an intravenous drug and involves a high risk of HIV/AIDS infection when using or sharing contaminated needles. (UN Office of Drugs and Crime, P. 19 Nov 2003).

The method of administering ATS depends on its preparation and varies from one place to the other. Taking it in tablet form or pills is the most common method in most South East Asian countries, especially China, Cambodia and Philippines.

A few countries, like Thailand, report an increased number of young people 'chasing the dragon' or inhaling the drug.

Young adult age groups use ATS as a form of recreation and for enjoyment, while others, especially night workers like truck drivers, nurses, miners, and security staff uses them to keep awake and work long hours. (ACCORD Report, November 2001, P 41).

Addiction, dependency, tolerance and craving of Amphetamine type stimulants is a much more expensive, powerful and deadly cycle than any other illicit drug.

ATS addicts are putting themselves at a very high risk of injury, such as physical disabilities, psychological disturbances, moral disorder and spiritual bankruptcy.

To make it much more worse, the treatment has so far been a failure and there is not much treatment or rehabilitation for ATS consumers and those that are addicted. Drug experts and professionals are yet to develop treatment methods and facilities to quickly to deal with the growing ATS problem.

The treatment methods and facilities for other drugs are quite different and its experiences are quite different and cannot be transferred or substituted for ATS treatment and rehabilitation. (UN Office of Drug and Crime, November, 2003).

The ATS epidemic is a completely new disaster that requires quick intervention programs and new anti-trafficking strategies that involve reduction skills and manpower. (UN Office of Drug and Crime, November 2003, p 19).

The international community, including government agencies, the NGOs and the churches have made calls to prevent and reduce the ATS supply by strengthening the control of precursors and identifying clandestine laboratories.

Cutting the supply line and the underground production of ATS in clandestine laboratories will reduce the demand. This is a very complex situation and risks are involved with criminal elements. (UN Office of Drugs and Crime, Update, November, 2003, p 9).

The ATS is a synthetic type of drug and it is divided into two major groupings:

1. Amphetamines (amphetamine and methamphetamine)

These types of drugs are very powerful and are addictive stimulants that concentrate on the brain biochemical system. They block the natural flow of the biochemical to the brain's central nervous system (CNS).
They also act as a depressant drug, which produce intense ups and downs creating real life dilemmas and devastating effects. (UN Office Drugs and Crime, November, 2003, P 19).

2. Ecstasy Type Substances (MDMA, MDA, MDE)

The Ecstasy Type Substances are synthetic drugs that cause deep mystical, physical, psychedelic and stimulant effects. It is known to cause coma, death from overdose and suicide.

It is also a multiple drug use or poly drug because it contains other substances of abuse. (UN Office of Drugs and Crime, November 2003, P 19).

Chapter 11

Inhalants and Their Abuse

INHALANT abuse is a relatively new and progressive problem affecting society, especially children and those who live under extreme poverty and suffer psychosocial problems. These people use inhalants to cope with life stresses. Sniffing solvent is a worldwide concern according to World Health Organisation reports.

The problem is complex because the substances that are being used are not illicit like other hard drugs.

Inhalant abuse was not common in PNG until recent times but the practice is spreading very fast among street kids. Buying and sniffing a tube of glue or contact cement is one of the most common forms of inhalant abuse in PNG.

There is no law against the use of these substances nor against other substances that people sniff, like petrol and varnish and so forth. Hundreds of these kinds of chemicals are openly sold over the counter and consumers are free to buy them for their authentic use.

We cannot make laws against the use of these products because they have special beneficial uses. For example, we cannot ban petrol because it is essential for running vehicles.

All that can be done is labelling the container or dispenser warning the general public of the dangers of inhaling the substance.

On the whole we are in a complex situation and we are not so sure what action to take.

The best option at the moment is for parents must be vigilant and ensure that their children are not getting involved in inhalant abuse.

1   Types of Inhalants

There are four (4) main types of inhalants namely **volatile solvents**, **gases**, **aerosols** and **nitrites**.

a.   Volatile solvents are liquids such as glue, gasoline, paint thinners and others.
b.   Gases, including medical gases .
c.   Aerosol sprays are prevalent inhalants in the homes and other common places. Hair and body sprays are two common examples.
d.   Nitrites are believed to stimulate sexual intercourse while the others alter moods.

2   Types of Substance

The substances that are used are found in stores, chemist shops, and other locations. They include sprays, paint, fresheners, insecticides, fingernail polish, kerosene and petrol.

3   The Common Inhalant Users

The common inhalant users are mostly problem kids and street kids who have no proper parental guidance and are at risk and most vulnerable to doing all sorts of things relating to drugs.

They use inhalants as a modern coping behaviour to deal with social and psychological stress and other difficulties in life. It gives them a false hope of relief from frustration, boredom, and rebellious against parents, guardians, teachers and authorities without knowing that they bring serious health risks.

The chemicals or substances the kids use are common and they are easy to find. For most it is a poor man's drug, meaning it is much cheaper and easier to find than other drugs. The inhaler feels high, confused, disoriented and often experiences hallucinations and paranoia.

4   The Effects on the Body

Inhalants act as a **depressant drug** slowing down the thinking process and making the inhaler feel depressed.

The user only experiences euphoria or good feelings for a short time. When his or her bodily functions and coordination is affected and the user acts intoxicated. His mind is out of control and cannot reason out things and he behaves improperly. He is confused, disoriented, fearful and experiences hallucinations and delusions. He can then become unconscious.

The user will often vomit and have bloodshot or radiant eyes. His heartbeat is slowed and he may even have heart failure.

The lungs may become poisoned and filled with the fumes and he may suffocate to death.

The long term results are damages to the brain and nervous system as well as the liver and kidneys.

If the user mixes both inhalant drugs and alcohol or any other drugs, the risk to his or her health is higher.

The fumes of the drug normally enters the blood stream very fast and circulates to all parts of the body within minutes, especially the brain and the liver where there is more blood circulation.

The central nervous system then depresses some bodily functions, including breathing and heartbeat.

The effects the drugs produce depend upon:

➢ The amount of chemicals being taken and absorbed i.e. whether the chemical has been inhaled once, moderately or several times.

➢ If it is taken on a regular basis with a short lapse of time in between.

➢ The age of the user, whether he is a child or a grown up person and his past experience in using the drug.

➢ The environment or conditions in which the inhaler uses the drug, for example, in an open space or in a confined room.

Body parts affected and how they are affected:

a. **The sensory or sense system**
    ➢ Sensitive to light
    ➢ Eye irritation
    ➢ Double vision and ringing in the ears

b. **The Lungs and the Heart**
    ➢ Difficulty in breathing
    ➢ Abnormal heart beat
    ➢ Chest pain

c. **The Stomach**
  - ➤ Nausea
  - ➤ Vomiting

Chapter 12

Alcohol

1   What is Alcohol?

ALCOHOL gets its meaning from the Arabic word *Al-kohol*, meaning a fine powder for colouring the eyebrows. It later became a term came to designate;

➢   A group of compounds that are used in industries or chemistry, usually additive solvents.

➢   A group of beverages containing ethyl alcohol.

The alcohol we drink is called ethanol (or ethyl alcohol), where yeast acting on carbohydrates in fruits and grains produce ethanol through fermentation or distillation.

Ethanol alcohol is composed of 2 carbon atoms, 5 hydrogen atoms, and a hydroxyl group.

2   Different Types of Alcohol

There are three common types of alcoholic beverage that people in PNG consume. They are;

1. **Beer**

   Beer, which is a common alcoholic beverage, is fermented from grains and fruits and contain 3 to 6 percent alcohol.

2. Wine

Wine is fermented from fruits. Ordinary wine contains 12 to 16 percent alcohol. Fortified wine has a core alcohol content with alcoholic percentage of 18 to 38.

3. Distilled Liquors

Distilled liquors are produced from distilled or heated-off alcohol and contain 36 to 65 percent alcohol content. It is often called degrees of proof. E.g. 80 proof liquor is 40 percent alcohol.

Some of these distilled liquors are gin, brandy, vodka, whiskey, and rum.

Alcoholic beverages are divided into those obtained by fermentation and those obtained by distillation.

	Beverage	Source	Alcohol Percentage
Fermentation	Beer	Malted Barley	3 to 6 percent
	Wine	Grapes	10 to 18 percent
Distillation	Whisky	Malted Grains	40 to 50 percent
	Brandy	Grapes	40 to 50 percent
	Rum	Molasses	40 to 50 percent
	Gin	Various	40 to 50 percent
	Vodka	Potatoes	50 to 60 percent

Alcohol drinks are made by fermentation of sugars from different natural substances like grain, fruit, cereal etc.

3 The effects of Alcohol

Alcohol can damage almost every part of the body. The worst damage occurs after years of abuse but even after a few drinks alcohol kills brain cells and changes the way you think, feel and act.

The effects of alcohol vary from person to person and depend on:

- ➤ The amount and rate at which it is consumed.
- ➤ The size and weight of the person (physical build).
- ➤ The health condition of the consumer.
- ➤ The occasion on which alcohol is consumed e.g. with a meal or just alone etc.
- ➤ Whether the alcohol is consumed with other drugs.
- ➤ Age and gender differences.

4 Immediate Effects

- ➤ Relaxation.
- ➤ Slurred speech.
- ➤ Aggression.
- ➤ Unconsciousness.
- ➤ Uncoordinated movements.
- ➤ Blurred vision.
- ➤ Dizziness.
- ➤ Slow reactions.
- ➤ Vomiting.
- ➤ Unclear judgment.

Continued drinking over a short period of time can cause a hangover, headache, nausea, shakiness and possibly vomiting.

5   Long Term Effects

➤ Poor diet.
➤ Memory loss or blackouts.
➤ Thinking is confused.
➤ Depression.
➤ Relationship problems.
➤ Poor work performance.
➤ Financial difficulties.
➤ Legal problems.
➤ Stomach inflammations.
➤ Frequent infections.
➤ Skin problems.
➤ Liver damage.
➤ Brain damage.
➤ Damage to reproductive organs.

6   Damage on Body Parts

❖ **The Brain**

Alcohol distorts the chemical messages that brain cells send to one another, which in a sober person enables him or her to think and act sensibly.

At first drinking can make you feel relaxed and sociable. But if drinking continues, your thoughts become jumbled and the brain centres governing speech, vision and balance do not function well.

When that happens the alcohol may cause you to;

➤ Become violent and start a fight.

> ➢ Lose control of a car and possibly kill someone.
> ➢ Wake up in a strange place and be unable to remember how you got there.
> ➢ Have sex when otherwise you wouldn't and possibly end up becoming pregnant, causing pregnancy or contracting a sexually transmitted disease such as AIDS.

Alcohol abuse can destroy parts of the brain, causing confusion, memory loss, thinking difficulties, unconsciousness and even death. While the brain is eroding so is the rest of the body.

❖ The Liver

The alcohol we drink enters the liver and the liver breaks it down by a chemical process using enzymes. The enzymes have to do extra work when alcohol enters the liver and this extra chemical reaction is called alcohol dehydrogenise.

Years of drinking causes scarring of the liver, which prevents the organ from performing its many vital functions.

Among other things, a scarred liver can no longer clean the blood of bodily poisons, which then injure other organs.

Excessive alcohol use can cause liver cirrhosis, which can result in death. The main effect of alcohol is on the liver cells. When liver cells die, scar tissue develops and cause fatty liver and liver hepatitis.

❖ The Pancreas

Alcohol can cause the lining of the pancreas to swell. The swelling can block off the passage from the pancreas to the small intestine.

Chemicals needed in the small intestine to aid digestion cannot get through. As a result, those chemicals begin to digest the pancreas itself causing abdominal pain, vomiting and possibly death.

❖ The Heart

Alcohol can increase the workload of the heart. Heavy use of alcohol over many years can damage the heart muscles. The heart tries to compensate for the damage by growing larger. But eventually it becomes unable to pump enough blood to meet the needs of the body resulting in other bodily complications.

Alcohol can also cause high blood pressure, which can damage the heart and cause irregular heartbeats.

❖ The Muscles

Alcohol can injure other muscles besides those in the heart. Heavy alcohol use may cause weakness by preventing muscle cells from absorbing calcium, which the muscle cells need to contract.

❖ The Stomach

Alcohol irritates the lining of the stomach and can cause vomiting. Excessive use of alcohol will cause stomach ulcers and haemorrhages of the stomach lining. Long term use of alcohol can lead into gastritis, which is an inflammation of the stomach lining and can cause stomach cancer.

❖ Alcohol and Pregnancy

Alcohol, like most other drugs crosses the placenta of the alcoholic mother and may affect the development of the unborn child resulting in various deformities. Drinking during pregnancy has been linked with higher risks of miscarriage and still and premature births.

Babies affected by alcohol may experience:

➢ Slower growth before and after birth.
➢ Prenatal weight deficiencies and low birth weight.
➢ Defects of the face, heart and other organs.
➢ Mental disabilities.
➢ Foetal alcohol syndrome (FAS).
➢ Cardiac dysfunction.

There is evidence that a glass of alcohol can affect a baby. The safest approach is not to drink at all during pregnancy.

Chapter 13

What is an Alcoholic?

THE following definition is from the World Health Organization and the Addiction Research Centre of Ontario in Canada.

"An alcoholic can be defined as any person whose consumption goes beyond the traditional and customary dietary user or the ordinary compliance with social drinking customs of the whole community .... a person with a chronic illness with certain identifiable characteristics, including continuing impairment of physical, emotional and occupational functioning as the direct result of alcohol use."

1   Definition of Alcoholism (Alcoholism as a Disease)

Disease criteria:

➢ Known aetiology.
➢ Known progression of symptoms.
➢ Known outcome (death).

According to the American Medical Society, "Alcoholism is a chronic, progressive and potentially fatal disease. It is characterized by tolerance and physical dependence, pathological changes or both, all direct consequences of the alcohol ingested".

Jellinek's Types of Alcoholism (Species).

> **Alpha alcoholism**: the earliest stage of the disease, manifesting the purely psychological continual dependence on the effects of alcohol to relieve bodily or emotional pain. This is the "problem drinker", whose drinking creates social and personal problems. While there are significant social and personal problems, these people can stop if they really want to.

> **Beta alcoholism**: polyneuropathy, or cirrhosis of the liver from alcohol without physical or psychological dependence. These are the heavy drinkers that drink a lot, almost every day. They do not have physical addiction and do not suffer withdrawal symptoms. This group do not have a "disease".

> **Gamma alcoholism**: involving acquired tissue tolerance, physical dependence, and loss of control. This is the alcoholic, who is very much out of control, and does have a "disease".

> **Delta alcoholism**: as in **Gamma alcoholism**, but with inability to abstain, instead of loss of control.

> **Epsilon alcoholism**: the most advanced stage of the disease, manifesting as dipsomania, or periodic alcoholism.

2   Dependence

Increased tolerance to alcohol may lead to physical and psychological dependency. At that point, alcohol becomes part of the person's normal physical and emotional functioning. Physical and psychological dependence is characterized by the presence of withdrawal symptoms when the use of drugs is discontinued suddenly.

Alcohol dependence is the presence of physical and psychological dependency and loss of control, some known factors are:

➢ Avoiding meals when drinking.
➢ Sneaking drinks.
➢ Drinking in the morning.
➢ Drinking before a party or occasion to get enough drinks.
➢ Constant blackouts when drinking.
➢ Drinking alone and don't want others to be around.
➢ Hiding drinks away from other people and don't want others to see it.
➢ Gulping drinks.
➢ More time is spent on drinking alcohol than other activities.
➢ Legal problems with police and courts for breaking of laws, like fighting with other people etc.
➢ Failure to carry out family obligations or responsibilities.
➢ Continuous family problems like violence at home and physical and emotional abuses.
➢ Hands shaking after drinking.
➢ Morning drinking to get rid of a hangover.
➢ Fear that one is an alcoholic.
➢ Promises to give up drinking but don't work out well.
➢ Sometimes heavy and continuous drinking after promising not to take anymore.
➢ Finding it difficult to give up drinking completely and instead becoming completely intoxicated.

(The Disease of Alcoholism by Dr. E.M. Jellinek).

3   The Addiction Process

Dr. W.K Van Dijk and Dr. E.M Jellinek did extensive work on the disease of alcoholism, including progressive charting of the addiction stages, and came up with the following four steps in the addiction process:

1.   Contact with the chemical or drug,
2.   Experimentation,
3.   Integrated use and
4.   Excessive use which leads into addiction.

4   The Definitions

"**Addiction** is seen as a disease of physical and psychological dependency which develops tolerance and craving."

"**Tolerance** is when the body gets so used to the drug or chemical and the need to increase the dose over and over again to feel the same effect."

"**Cross tolerance** is when someone is tolerant to one form of drug can also be tolerant to another drug." E.g. Alcohol and Cocaine.

"**Craving** is a powerful and forceful drive and motivating factor in drinking. You cannot just stop it, there is a real need, the body needs it, and you can't stop thinking of taking alcohol. Craving is a reinforcer with uncontrollable and compulsive drinking behaviour. Craving makes you a slave and all your morals are gone and you are controlled by something else."

5   The Physiological Dependence

The cellular adjustment to chemical intake has already been set up and the body gets used to the drug and becomes tolerant to the chemical. When the chemical intake is stopped completely, the life threatening disease known as withdrawal symptoms is then developed. More and more drugs are taken to feel the same effect.

6   The Psychological Dependence

The thinking process is already set up or converted to taking in more and more of the chemical or craving for increased chemical intake.

Those people who have experienced social and psychological problems like depression, discomfort, paranoia, shame, guilt, marital problems, rejection, fear and etc. are more prone to take more and more chemicals that lead to the disease of addiction. They take drugs as a modern coping behaviour to control tensions and escape from reality or real problems.

The most common behaviours associated with psychological dependency is the level of ego defence, denial, rationalisation, minimization, intellectualization, projection etc. Their chemical dependence is constantly maintained by their psychological ego defence mechanisms.

7   Withdrawal Symptoms

When alcohol or drug intake is discontinued or stopped, withdrawal symptoms take effect. The alcoholic or drug addict becomes physically and emotionally ill.

Alcoholism and drug addiction are diseases with no known cures and stopping them will add another problem of withdrawal symptoms - there is no middle road.

8   The Stages of Addiction

Van Dijk defined four stages of addiction which include:

1. **Progressive** - contact with the chemical. The chemical is easily assessable and available.
2. **Chronic** - experiment or want to taste the drug out of curiosity. Often the new comer would want to taste the chemical and feel good.
3. **Foetal** - excessive use of chemical due to psychological and physiological factors.
4. **Primary use** - addiction develops which is life threatening and dangerous. Withdrawal symptoms are set up when the chemical is discontinued.

Chapter 14

More On The Disease of Alcoholism

WHY some people become alcoholics and others do not depends on their personality, environmental factors, social factors, psychological factors, genetic factors, moral and spiritual factors and approach to drinking. They all contribute towards the disease of alcoholism.

An alcoholic person can be recognized and can be helped successfully if he admits his problems. He can live a normal life if he stops drinking completely. There are two things an alcoholic must do in order to stay sober.

❖ He is recognized as an alcoholic person who needs treatment and
❖ He accepts this fact himself.

The sooner he is recognized as an alcoholic the better his chances of recovery.

How can we recognize the signs and symptoms of alcoholism from the early stage to the progressive and final stages?

1. The Early Stage Which Is Called Prodromal Stage

When we get malaria we feel our body get weaker. We feel cold and shiver and want to stay close to the fire. Then we get hot and throw off our blankets. Foods are tasteless. We feel dizzy and don't feel like doing anything. Then we know immediately that we have malaria because these are the signs and symptoms of malaria.

It happens in a similar way to an alcoholic person. The early signs are that the drinker drinks to feel joy and this joy hooks him and he wants to explore further.

He discovers that he finds relief and happiness and the feeling of being a nobody is replaced by feeling of being someone of great status. He feels no shame, no fear and is confident talking to girls. He feels important and one with the world. He suffers from hangovers and naturally wants to feel such pleasant feelings again so he resorts to drinking again more often.

During this period the drinker changes his personality and behaviour. None-talkers become talkative and a friendly person becomes aggressive and wants to fight. If he drinks heavily enough very often there is no hangover the next day.

2.   <u>First Stage</u>

One morning the alcoholic person wakes up to realize that his drinking pattern has suffered a change. He cannot remember what happened while he was drinking the night before.

He did not faint or fall unconscious or go to sleep during this time. He did normal things and appeared normal but he has no memory of the events and people around him from the night before. He cannot remember them. He experiences a complete loss of memory or what is called blackout. This is a frightening experience for the drinker.

At this time the alcoholic not only drinks for enjoyment as before but also to drown his fears and restore his confidence. Instead of drinking slowly he drinks quickly to feel the same effect sooner.

During this time he may begin to hide how much he drinks and sneaks extra before going to a party. It may mean he drinks on his way. He will make sure he has alcohol every time in any location, either at sports, public gatherings and at meetings or on trips.

During this first stage, the alcoholic realises that something no good is happening to his drinking. He cannot forget drinking even though sometimes he wishes he could give up. When his wife tells him about his drinking habits, he tells her to stop nagging and leave him alone.

3.   Second (Crossroad/Crucial) Stage

This stage means loss of control in drinking. This is crossroad. This road is always a journey downhill and the alcoholic will never return back to social drinking like other people do.

Loss of control means getting drunk when he does not want to do so or against his will. Once the alcoholic has reached this stage, he should never drink again.

However, to tell him to stop drinking or cut down is like telling a person with a bad cold to stop coughing. He cannot drink less.

He can quit drinking entirely but he cannot drink just a little. Once he starts drinking the alcohol becomes his boss and he drinks until he is intoxicated or drunk and the beer is all gone and all the money is spent.

It is at this stage of the illness that the alcoholic has the guiltiest feelings. He is often ashamed of what he does while drinking and feels remorse or bad about it.

And he does the same thing over and over again the next time he drinks. To forget or hide his shame, he may act like a big man while drinking, talking big, giving orders and supplying drinks to anyone around him.

Usually at about this time a crisis may occur, such as road accident, falling down the steps or forgetting an important assignment or getting fired. This brings shock to the alcoholic and he decides to do something about his drinking.

He either:

➢ Change his drinking pattern, e.g. drinking only at certain times such as only at weekends.
➢ He tries to quit alcohol entirely.

All those attempts are doomed to fail. He will drink out of control again, worse than ever.

Dr. Jellinek says that all his researches points to the fact that a change in drinking pattern is the strongest sign of the downward course of the disease.

When those attempts fail, the alcoholic may try moving to a different place, for example, moving to another town, taking another job, or going back to his village. However, he takes the disease with him wherever he goes and whatever he does. His drinking still remains out of control.

At this time, the alcoholic's fear of not having alcohol is so great that he tries all kinds of things to protect his supply of it. Well-meaning relatives and friends may try to keep him from drinking and so with all the cleverness at his command he will try to fool them. You cannot imagine all the places in which an alcoholic can hide his bottles.

A common problem at this time is losing sexual power. The alcoholic who has used alcohol in the past to increase his sexual power now realises that he is losing his strength and is frightened.

He does not realise that it is the alcohol that has weakened his ability to have sex and so he drinks more to recover it. He may sleep with other women to prove that he is as strong as ever.

This not only makes his wife get suspicious and angry but after a while he begins to think that his wife is playing around with other men just as he is playing around with other women and soon he is accusing her of doing what he is doing.

Physically, the alcoholic is now shaky, nervous and often feels liking throwing up. He therefore skips breakfast and cannot face the day without his morning drink or eye opener.

Another mark has been reached and that is drinking taking the place of eating and as a result, malnutrition and physical decay set in. He complains of extreme tiredness and may appear to the doctor as being 'sick and tired'.

4.   Important Signs of Second (Crossroads/Crucial) Stage

➢   Loss of control of drinking.
➢   Making excuses or rationalization.
➢   Acting as a big man while drinking.
➢   Changes often from showing regret to anger.
➢   Always secretly ashamed.
➢   Quits drinking for a period of time.

> ➢ Tries to change his drinking habits.
> ➢ Begins losing friends who don't drink like he does.
> ➢ Leaves or loses jobs.
> ➢ Loses interest in things not connected with drinking.
> ➢ Thinks about running away to escape his problems.
> ➢ Often angry for no good reason and resents other people.
> ➢ Protects his supply of alcohol.
> ➢ Often feels very sorry for himself
> ➢ Suffers malnutrition because of drinking instead of eating.
> ➢ May get very sick.
> ➢ Loses sexual desire and power.
> ➢ Unreasonable jealously of his wife.
> ➢ The morning drink.
> ➢ Directly goes to a medical clinic or doctor.
> ➢ Thinking more and more about drinking.
> ➢ Neglects his responsibilities.
> ➢ May have long periods of drinking and drunkenness.
> ➢ His family scolds him for his drinking.
> ➢ May lose his sense of time.
> ➢ His drinking causes the family to change their habits.
> ➢ He runs away or moves his home.

5.   **The Chronic And Final Stage; Constant**

This final stage of alcoholism is when the alcoholic can no longer hide himself and his problems are exposed to all to see. The times between drunkenness become shorter and the drinking lasts longer, often up to days at a time

The last bit of pretence and self-respect are gone. If his family has not gone by now, they probably will. And he seeks the company of poor people and other alcoholics with whom he feels no sense of shame or blame.

He will drink anything from home brew to methylated spirits, shaving lotion or anything that contains alcohol and he will beg, steal and borrow money to get it.

Physically, spiritually and mentally exhausted, he has really reached rock bottom. He loses tolerance for alcohol and gets drunk at every time possible.

However, unless his brain is too damaged, there is still hope that with his true cooperation treatment can restore him to health.

6. <u>Other Effects of Alcohol on the Body</u>

❖ The Brain

THE human brain is a complex cognitive control centre and the most important organ of a human being and is distinct from lower animals. It is composed of a higher faculty pertaining to the human mind which controls the behaviour, the personality and all other characteristics.

The human mind is often referred to as rational soul which processes intellect; the power to think, plan, learn new things, create and memorise things; control the movement of our bodies, behaviour and many other functions. It is capable of creating new things, gaining knowledge and doing complicated things.

All human beings have a thinking mind, the working mind and the reasoning faculty. Philosophers including the philosopher Immanuel Kant, regarded the mind as the core of human existence. (Encyclopaedia, Oxford Scientific Films, London).

With alcohol we are talking about a drug that impairs the brain mechanism, the psycho-motor performances, inhibits short term memory, blocks perception, slows down or affects learning process, reaction to time, impairs visual tracking, affects memory, causes panic, fear of dying, personality disorders and paranoid ideas. Increased doses causes hallucinations, i.e. seeing things and hearing voices or feeling things in their bodies that are not there or do not exist. (Dr. Gabriel Nahas, Queensland Health Depart report, 1991).

The human brain is divided into many complex sections each with its distinct functions and roles. The main sections in the brain are the cerebrum or frontal lobe/parietal lobe, cerebellum and brain stem. Components in the brain stem are medulla oblongata and the thalamus.

The cerebrum activates intelligence and reasoning power, controls behaviour and bodily movement and balance. The medulla controls breathing, blood circulation, heart rate, liver functioning and the movement of the body.

The thalamus sends chemicals or electrical messages to and from the cerebral cortex to all parts of the body. These are often called neurotransmitters. (Microsoft Encarta Encyclopaedia, Oxford Scientific Films/Landon).

One of the most important parts of human brain is the memory that stores layers of information like a recorder and data processor. It can analyse and view things of the past and the present with the hope of getting insights working towards the future.

Our intelligence depends on our memory i.e. how we remember things and memorise them correctly in exams or in our daily interactions.

Our emotions and feelings including pain, anger, fear, guilt, shame, remorse, sadness, happiness, gladness, excitement and others are activated from our memory.

Chapter 15

Risk Factors Known as Theories
of Causality and Alcohol

THERE has been a lot more research work in the field of alcoholism to determine whether alcoholism is a disease or not and it begins with Alcoholics Anonymous around 1957.

The American Medical Association declared alcoholism as a disease based on the logic: "that a disease has a known aetiology, a known progression of symptoms that get worse rapidly and an outcome and alcoholism fits well into those criteria."

The spread of alcohol abuse is getting worse in PNG and its aetiology, or study of its causes, to understand its prevalence, and to work out proper preventive measures, demand reduction, medical treatment, rehabilitation, healing and recovery has not been developed very far yet.

Sometimes we regard alcohol and drug problems as normal, ordinary and insignificant social problems that we can cope with or just ignore it.

Sometimes we realise it's a problem but we don't know how to handle it because we don't have the skills, knowledge, expertise and facilities, so we just ignore it. We don't even know where to refer alcoholics to for assistance because it's a disease that many of us are not aware of.

Medical treatment, rehabilitation, counselling and recovery from alcoholism and drug addiction is a long and tedious process requiring time, specialists, resources, commitment and personal willpower and responsibility. (Refer Dr. Jellinek's Stages of Addiction and Recovery).

Some people will say that chemical addiction is a bio-medical disease so doctors and nurses are to give addicts treatment at the hospital.

Others will say it's a law and order problem where policemen, courts and lawyers can handle it by putting the drug addicts into police custody and prison.

 Yet others will say, it's a moral and spiritual problem and those who consume drugs are sinners who are controlled by the devil and they need to go to a priest or pastor for spiritual guidance.

Still others will say it's a behavioural or attitude problem and only human scientists like psychologists, psychiatrists, social workers and counsellors can handle it by psycho-therapy or by sending alcoholics to psychiatric institutions for mental treatment and rehabilitation.

The alcohol and drug problem is quite different from other diseases and is a sort of **microcosm** with inter-connected or interrelated problems, each interacting or supporting the other.

There are many causes and effects including physical, psychological, emotional, social, spiritual, moral, legal and environmental aspects. Too assist a person to recover from alcoholism or drug addiction we have to look at all aspects and provide holistic preventive and treatment measures.

The term "the theories of casualties" (risk factors) classify four main areas requiring attention and as describes, specific assistance that will clearly define the sort of problems and the kind of assistance required. The four major theories of casualties or risk factors for the prevention and treatment of alcoholism and drug addiction are **biological/medical** theories, **psychological** theories, **sociological** theories and **spiritual/moral** theories.

1   The Biological/Medical Theories

Alcoholism is seen as a disease or symptom of bodily dysfunction or disturbances in the bodily structure, including brain damage, liver cirrhosis, heart disease, blood vesicles, nerve system, damages to the reproductive organs, cardiovascular disease, physical addiction and craving.

Physical addiction, dependency, tolerance and craving are seen as a genetic disease or disorder inherited by the young ones from their parents.

 The drug addict goes through severe brain damage and bodily disorder and his normal brain function is greatly affected.

A. The Model Perspectives

Since it is a disease like any other sickness, the care, treatment and responsibility of alcoholics and drug addicts belongs to medical workers, including psychiatrists, doctors and nurses. Patients are treated at the hospital with normal referrals and interviews, diagnosis, drug prescriptions as the addict goes through medical rehabilitation.

This medical rehabilitation and treatment is called **detoxification** and is where alcoholics and drug addicts are normally admitted and are on treatments under prudent medical administration until discharged or terminated.

This sort of treatment is well set up in developed countries with facilities, specialist doctors, psychologist, psychiatrist and counsellors to deal with.

Hospitals in PNG do not have detoxification units and we are yet to establish one at our hospitals with specialist doctors and nurses to treat addicts separately.

B. The Theories

(1) The Genetic Disorder

An inherited biochemical abnormality is the main factor or cause in excessive drinking or drug use according to some experts in the field of medicine and addiction.

The disease of drug addiction is seen as a hereditary disease passed on from the parents to their children. Once a father or mother is an alcoholic or a drug addict the child will also stand a high chance of becoming addicted to alcohol and drugs. While the pre-conditioning is already setup if he or she does not drink or take drugs it will not affect them.

(2) Brain Damage

Alcohol and drug consumption affects the brain and brain cells are destroyed.

The centre of the brain coordination and the mechanical system that controls the body are affected and do not function well.

Excessive use of alcohol causes severe brain damage and a

disorder known as **Korsakov syndrome**.

Thousands of brain cells are destroyed by continuous intake of alcohol and the brain becomes stupefied. Both short and long term memory are affected. Bodily coordination from the brain to the other parts of the body is affected. The brain nerve cells or neurons are affected. The brain chemical messages or receptors known as neurotransmitters are affected or disturbed when drug chemicals especially tetrahydrocannabinol (THC) blocks the spaces between the brain cells.

(3) The Endocrinological

Glandular disorders occur and nerve cells are destroyed. There are shaky hands when nerve cells are dead or not working properly. Shaky hands normally appear in alcoholics.

(4) The Other Medical Complications

Allergic reaction, addiction to food elements, eating disorders causing **anorexia** and **bulimia** are other complications that resemble the physiological and psychological problems.

Substance abuse leads to reduction of biological or bodily needs such as hunger, thirst, sleep, rest and sex.

2 The Psychological Model/Theories

There are multiple reasons why people resort to alcohol and drugs. Chemical dependency serves some purposes for the alcoholic or drug addicts to function normally.

There are reasons and motives that vary between different people, personality type, timing and physical and social environment or social conditions.

It could be psychological discomfort, loneliness, rejection, depression, work pressure or any other reason.

Chemical abuse and dependency is seen as a learned behaviour pattern. People learn to do things from observing or taking part.

The effects of drugs produces stress, depression, anxiety, hallucinations, delusions, memory loss, learning ability disorientation and psychosomatic illnesses. Drug abuse brings interpersonal problems, unconsciousness, dependency and cravings.

A. The Model Perspectives

- ➤ Drug abuse is seen as a coping behaviour for controlling tensions or serving some other purpose in life. People drink and take drugs because they are depressed, worried or are ashamed etc.

- ➤ The desire or degree of use varies from person to person. Some use more and others less. Excessive alcohol and drug use affects physical, psychological, mental, emotional, social and spiritual life and causes permanent damage.

- ➤ Alcohol and drug addiction are conditional behaviour patterns. The addict's psychological or emotional condition allows him or her to drink or take drugs.

B. The Theories

Alcohol and drug abuse produces known psychological effects including depression, anxiety, aggressiveness, memory lost, blackout, experience hallucinations, loss of interest and behavioural problems etc.

C. Learning Orientation

Some behaviours are learned from observing others doing it and are thus reinforced. People drink or take drugs by observing and also doing it out of curiosity and experimenting with it.

D. Social Learning/Environmental stress effects

In some settings the availability of drugs and the addictive and social behaviour of the people contribute to social learning. People live and do things in a sub-culture of addictive behaviour or personalities.

In the social environmental setting where alcohol and drugs are readily available and freely accessible, people learn to cope with it or be part of the problem.

E. Transactional Analysis

Eric Berne, an American Cognitive Psychologist formulated his psychological theory called **Transactional Analysis** and his popular study is called **Games Analysis**. He describes alcoholism as purely a social transaction involving two or more people in an alcoholic game.

This has nothing to do with biochemical and medical problems associated with alcoholism that only medical professionals can handle it. (Eric Berne – Games People Play, 1964)

Eric Berne explains five key game players in the **alcoholic game.** The game is played by mostly family members, including wives, mothers, fathers, children and other significant relations.

The alcoholic or drug addict himself is the **chief game player** and the other main supporting role is played by the wife or husband, who normally becomes the **prosecutor** who accuses the alcoholic over the drunkenness or addiction. Another role player is called the **rescuer,** normally a family friend who comforts the alcoholic, gives good advice, money, food and so on.

Another role player is called the **patsy,** which is normally played by the alcoholic's mother who provides comfort, gives food, and money and accuses the spouse of understanding the alcoholic.

Just take one drink only is another form of game, mostly played by best friends. Instead of getting one drink the alcoholic ends up getting intoxicated. (Eric Berne – Games People Play, 1964).

In group therapy transactional analysis is used with its special wordings but in a different context. This is based on the theory that people are meant to change their behaviours. They go through the process of personal growth and feelings of self-worth and they come to understand and admit their self-defeating characters through therapy sessions.

Once they come to grief with their problems and admit them they are allowing themselves to be free to experience personal growth, freedom to achieve sobriety and live a happy life. The main purpose of this therapy session is to build high self-esteem and make them feel okay. (Eric Berne – Games people Play, 1964).

Another term used and developed by Eric Berne and further modified by Harris is known as **the four life positions of human relations**.

a.   I am Ok and You are Ok.

This is a healthy life position where all people are important and equal and have respect for each other despite creed, colour, status and nationality.

b.   I am Ok and You are Not Ok.

This is a manipulative position where the alcoholic or drug addict considered himself to be important and special. He is the boss who is in control and people are to follow his advice and if they don't he fights them and gets rid of them. The alcoholic or drug addict thinks that he is always right and the rest are not and they have problems with alcohol and drugs but he is okay and others are not okay.

c.   I am Not Ok and You are Not Ok.

This position is completely unhealthy. Everybody is not okay. We are all losers, failures and unworthy. The alcoholic may   say, "You are useless and I am also useless." You are a drug   body and I am also a drug body. You are rubbish and I am also rubbish and the list goes on.

d.   I am Not Ok and You are Ok.

This position is unhealthy. The alcoholic considers himself unimportant, useless, stupid, ignorant, poor, criminal, helpless and unworthy etc. He thinks that all the rest are alright and he is not that good. I am not okay because I take drugs and homebrew.

These positions are not something new but are behaviours within us all that need to be acknowledged so we are aware of our positions in real life situations and can work towards making okay by respecting each other, taking responsibility, developing self-esteem, thinking positively, doing good things, avoiding doing bad things, correcting mistakes and respecting human values etc.

F.   Psychoanalytic Theory

1.   Unconscious Needs/Desires

The pioneer work of Sigmund Freud was centred around the unconscious part of our personality to uncover the hidden but valuable knowledge of self. What we know of in the conscious part of our lives through the senses is just the tip of the iceberg according to Freund. He said that if we dig deeper into our unconscious level of self we will discover buried emotions and suppressions of enormous magnitude that causes problems.

He further said that most of our emotions are recorded and stored in the unconscious side of our self and cannot be recalled except through self-awareness and exploration into the past. This makes us conscious of what is wrong and right and good and bad within us. (Nancy Chodorow, Psychoanalysis and the Sociology of Gender, 1978).

Freud said that the mind is divided into three levels, which included the **conscious, preconscious and the unconscious.**

➢ The conscious mind includes everything that we are aware of involving our five senses of seeing, feeling, hearing, smelling and tasting. This section of our mind allows us to think and act. It also includes our memory, which can process and store data and information. It can also link up with the preconscious.

➢ The preconscious mind is the component of the mind that

deals with our ordinary memory and can be brought back into consciousness at any time or in any situation. Sometimes we experience this as flash backs or the recalling of past experiences.

➤ The unconscious mind is the reservoir of psycho-energy and feelings, emotions, thoughts, urges and memories of our conscious awareness that are unacceptable or unpleasant, such as the feeling of pain, anxiety and conflict. Past painful experiences that are suppressed can also be recalled into consciousness as flash backs.

G. Personality Types

Carl Jung was an analytical psychologist who developed the theories of personality type known as **introverted** and **extraverted** personality.

Introverted people are quiet, live in isolation, keep to themselves, do not want other people to know them, do not socialise with others and are not interested in their ideas.

Extraverted people are open to others, share ideas, keep no secrets, socialise with others and are mostly people oriented. This personality type was further developed by M Briggs as a personality type indicator where people are categorised under 16 different types of personalities by answering carefully analysed questions to determine the different types.

H. Dreams and Self Awareness

Both Freud and Jung refer to dreams as **a road map to unconsciousness,** revealing some hidden parts of our knowledge that is repressed and suppressed. Sometimes we see the darker sides of our lives and other times the good sides of ourselves in dreams. They thought that the buried and hidden parts of lives are often revealed in dreams. Within the dreams there signs and symbols that reveal some sacred meanings of life.

Dreams and imaginations are important in human life and play an important role in our personal and spiritual growth. Scientists, philosophers, writers, musicians and even politicians when formulating scientific theories or getting their noble insights and ideas often contemplate these in their dreams and imaginations during sleep.

Increased knowledge in human science has made us aware that if each one of us wants to better understand ourselves then we need to increase our self-awareness and examine and tune into our inner messages. For example, when we feel lonely and are depressed we can try to do away with this unpleasant feeling by playing music or doing something else to divert our attention.

Our psycho-energy is released through biological means known as drives. A drive has two parts, a biological need and a psychological need. One of the most powerful drives is our sex drive, a strong physical desire to have sex and the psychological need to have sex to release the desire.

I. Freudian Personality Structures

➢ The Id

The id is the pleasure principle that tries to satisfy instinctual needs unconsciously. It is everything that is psychological that is inherited, including our instinct for survival and reservoirs of psycho energy.

The id represents our inner world of subjective experience and has no knowledge of objective reality. Sexual pleasure derives from the id.

➢ The Ego

The ego deals with our rational thinking and planning. The ego is the executive or the manager of our personality because it controls the reasons for our actions, selects the features of our environment to which it will respond and decides what instincts will be satisfied and in what manner. The ego tries to protect itself against undue anxiety and moral anxiety. The ego is concerned about the reality of things.

➢ The Superego

The superego deals with the internalized standards of society involved with psychological rewards of pride and self-love but also punishment, involving guilt, shame, fear and inferiority complex problems.

The superego is composed of two parts, the conscious and self-esteem. It strives for the ideal rather than the real and strives for perfection, which is reinforced by the rewards and punishments.

The superego is like the parental voice that strives for perfection. The superego is the code of conduct within us, offering choices between good and bad, right or wrong, value or dis-value, worth or un-worth etc.

J.   Alcoholic and/or Drug User Personality Types

❖ Low Frustration Tolerance

The alcoholic or drug addict is impatient and experiences uncomfortable and uneasy feelings in a situation. The alcoholic or drug addict experiences uncontrolled depression, anger, feelings of guilt, shame, fear, resentment and anxiety.

❖ **Anxiety**

All human beings experience anxiety at certain stages of their life but to alcoholics and drug addicts it's much worse. It is called **free float anxiety** and the addicts lives in constant fear that forces him or her to create problems and then run away from them. Unforeseen happenings pop up simultaneously or without warning.

❖ **Grandiosity**

The alcoholic or the drug addict uses his or her drinking behaviour as protective armour to hide his or her low self-esteem or inferiority complex problems. He or she feels useless, unworthy, inadequate and defeated so he or she escapes by drinking to hide his or her true feelings. Drinking is seen as a shield to protect himself or herself from others e.g. a quiet person becomes talkative and acts big when he or she is drunk.

❖ **Perfectionism**

Alcoholics and the drug addicts set up impossible goals but never follow through, resulting in failure. The alcoholic sees themselves as an idealist with creative ideas that are never fulfilled. They often talk about impossible things that they will never achieve.

Sometimes, as we have seen, alcoholics or drug addicts are intelligent and can deal with complex issues which no normal person can comprehend or understand.

Where alcoholics and addicts are creative they only become successful when they give up their drinking.

Wishful Thinking

Even though all of us experience wishful thinking, alcoholics and drug addicts can take this to another level. Alcoholics interpret their dreams as something real that has happened or is going to happen. An alcoholic will say that he or she will be a business man or women soon, buying a car, a building and shares in companies and so forth. However, in reality they are just another poor hapless human being.

❖ **Isolation**

Alcoholics and the drug addicts are living in isolation and do not want to socialise or be with others except their own drinking mates and peers. At times they drink in isolation and don't want others to know about it or see them. A worker might drink in the office alone hiding from others.

❖ **Sensitivity**

This exaggerates all the unpleasant feelings, hatred, resentment, anger, fears, guilt, hurt and shame towards others until the alcoholic feels really down and helpless. They drink and take drugs to escape from unpleasant feelings. For example, a woman might drink as relief from hurt and frustration after her husband has deserted her for no good reason.

❖ **Impulsiveness**

I want what I want whenever I want it. This is related to **low frustration tolerance** that all alcoholics and addicts seem to have. In some ways the alcoholic or drug addict takes a certain pride in this impulsiveness as though it was a valuable asset. He does not enjoy a job or task given to him. He wants to finish it quickly and becomes frustrated. He only works at what he wants until the fun is gone.

❖ Defiance

Defiance is a characteristic of criminal behaviour that conflicts with the law and society. The alcoholic or drug addict feels rejected from the society and the society also rejects him or her because he or she cannot fit in well as a moral being who can contribute meaningfully to it.

Defiant alcoholics or drug addicts are people who develop a tendency for fighting and destroying properties, grabbing things from others and making themselves look like heroes.

❖ Dependence

Dependence on another person or persons is common in all alcoholics and drug addicts. They cannot support themselves and depend on others for their daily living. An addict has no money but begs from others to support his or her habits.

3   Sociological/Environmental Model/Theories

1.   Model Perspectives

➢ Social, economic and environmental conditions determine the level and use of drugs.

➢ Nature means heredity and nurture means environment which influences and contributes enormously to alcoholism and addiction diseases and problems.

➢ Relationship between social structure, social stratification and prevalence of alcoholism and drug abuse.

➢ Importance of association with various social and cultural groups.

2. Theories

❖ Cultural

Cultural attitudes and degree of tensions. In the cultural setting where alcohol is served as normal drinks in parties, bride price exchange, birth day parties etc., the success of the party depends on how many cartons of beer one buys and consumes.

In some cultural settings drinking alcohol or taking drugs is prohibited and there is less people involved in taking alcohol or drugs. There is less abusive drinking because of strong cultural values and respect for community laws.

❖ Sub-Cultural

Social conditioning, social variables, external triggers and social cohesion. Human beings are continuously exposed and influenced by other people and the social environment they live in.

If normal people are being exposed to the predominately alcohol or drug oriented culture and environment they are continuously forced to take in alcohol and drugs. They lived under social pressure and influences of negative behaviour and drinking pattern.

Peer pressure is more strong in our culture and peer pressure towards drinking adds more drinking problems than any other causes. Someone out of respect will force you to take one drink only but instead of taking one you end up getting drunk.

3. Deviant Behaviour

❖ Part of Pattern of Deviance

Deviant behaviour is defined as someone behaving and doing things contrary or outside the moral and ethical guidelines or standard of rules in a given society. Deviants are people who break rules and often act abnormal. They are real manipulators in conning others, telling lies, cheating, displaying aggressiveness, violent behaviours, stealing and etc. to support their deviant behaviour. Deviant people continuously involve themselves in crimes because they cannot know the difference between right and wrong, good and bad, lawful and unlawful, moral and immoral and etc.

4   Morality/Ethics and Spiritual Models

1. Model Perspectives

➢ Our behaviour is based on spiritual, ethical or moral values or what is judged good or bad, rightful and wrongful, sinful or not sinful, value or not value etc...

➢ Acceptable or unacceptable behaviour is based on universally accepted morality or principle of doing good and avoiding evil.

➢ These models place emphasis on the harm within the chemical substance.

➢ Use and abuse of drugs is seen as wrong, sinful and illegal because it destroys human beings affecting their moral and spiritual growth.

➤ People, including alcoholics and drug addicts are special because they are created in the image of God and the immortality of their soul or life after dead (Parousia).

➤ Chemical abuse is seen as relating to unmet spiritual and moral needs such as;

❖ **Faith**

Alcoholics and drug addicts began to lose faith in their religion or high power because their lives are unmanageable. Their personal relationship with God, the life of prayer, meditation and spirituality fades.

❖ **Hope**

As Christians we have hope for the future and try to be good and spiritual and believe in life after death. Alcoholics and drug addicts lose hope in their future and they feel hopeless and really don't know where they are going.

❖ **Love**

Alcoholics and drug addicts will not show any love or concern towards fellow human beings and show no reverence to God as their creator. The only love known to them is selfish erotic love, decorated with sexual pleasure.

❖ **Forgiveness**

There is no sense of forgiveness among alcoholics and drug addicts. It is too difficult for them to forgive others who have done wrong to them. Only brave people have the courage and strength to do so.

❖ Serenity

Alcoholics and drug addicts are not living in peace and harmony with their fellow human beings and God. Their minds are bombarded with conflict and problems and are scattered. There is no serenity or inner peace among alcoholics and drug addicts..

❖ Humanity

Alcoholics and drug addicts do not feel like humans who have values or have respect for others or treat them as equals.

❖ Humility

Alcoholics and drug addicts cannot be humble in the presence of others. They feel that they are special and look down on others.

❖ Justice

There is no sense of justice among alcoholics and drug addicts. They create injustices for their families by not supporting them financially.

❖ Equality

Alcoholics and drug addicts don't see other human beings as equals with the same dignity and value as persons who are created in the image of God.

❖ Truth

Alcoholics and drug addicts normally tell lies and there is no need for the truth in them.

❖ Sincerity

Chemical abusers are not sincere and honest to themselves.

❖ Spirituality

Spirituality affects all men and women. People are not free but become slaves to drugs, a non- living material that blocks good moral choices. When human beings are free from all forms of problems they are enriched in spirit and progress towards inner peace and perfection.

Chapter 16

Counselling, Treatment & Rehabilitation

1   Adolescence Drug Counselling

CARL ROGERS is a humanist psychologist and he believes that human beings have the potential and inner strength to change their behaviours and attitudes. Human beings are gifted with enormous powers to overcome psychological blockages that stop them from growing as their authentic selves.

A counsellor can facilitate behaviour change processes but it is the responsibility of the client to change and grow.

We are now in a complex situation in PNG where there are rapid social changes being brought about by modernisation. This has created deeply rooted psychological problems, social and economic pressures, frustrations, rebellion against parents and authorities and, emerging genetic disorders.

PNG youths living in the transitional phase between childhood and adolescence are particularly vulnerable. Where once we as parents and guardians could control our children's behaviour with rules, regulations, cultural norms and values this is becoming increasingly more difficult. The youths are being exposed to the influences of a confused adult world due to these social changes.

We cannot do much as this becomes part of their norm and sub-culture so we have to cope with it hoping that they don't get worse. Drugs and alcohol are key elements in these new changes.

The goal of counselling is to help motivate and enable drug addicts and alcoholics to change their behaviour and return to normal life. The addict has to free himself or herself from past mistakes and painful experiences with drugs, alcohol abuse, emotional difficulties, depression, anxiety and bad interpersonal relationships and find a constructive means and ways of dealing with life situations.

Counselling involves an emphatic and genuine relationship between the counsellor and the client and is one based on real life experiences, perceptions and awareness.

A counselling relationship is built on trust, respect, understanding and concern for others. Counselling should be oriented towards achieving goals and should explore unresolved hidden social and psychological influences that stop personal growth.

Through genuine support and a warm relationship the addict can then gain confidence and trust and becomes free to handle problems and progress towards life adjustment. The addict comes to a full realisation of his or her value and their potential in personal growth, education and a professional career.

There are many counselling theories and characteristics but it is important to base our counselling on a holistic method like the **eclectic therapy model**, which takes from bits and pieces of various counselling theories, techniques and methods of counselling to adapt them to the specific needs of individual clients, including their cultural and social situations and conditions and the nature of their problems.

According to Grunebaum and Chasin "the adolescent drug addict is seen from three different perspectives: **historical, interaction** and **experiential**. Treatment is based on three approaches – **"understanding, transformation (changes) and identification"** (Chasin and Grunebaum, 1982).

For **understanding the counsellor** observes, identifies, interacts, probes and fosters intimate discloser in order to assist the client's knowledge on the nature and origin of his or her drug problems.

The first step is to recognise the problem, the root causes and contributing factors in order to assist the client to come to realise the problems in their present forms.

To enable **transformation** the counsellor systematically directs the client in order to modify and correct dysfunctional behaviours and attitudes and move towards achieving sobriety. The counsellor assists the client in identifying problems and practical steps to motivate his transformation or change of behaviour.

For **identification**, the counsellor acts on an example (living model) designing and taking part in emotional experience. (Chasin and Grunebaum, 1982).

The goal of counselling is to promote a new identity and discover what is healthy and true within the individual. In order to change to become a healthy person the addict must recognise his or her inner psychological conflicts.

According to Loevinger those three approaches are equivalent to child rearing and to the way children learn in a kindergarten. "Parents tend to rear children either by explaining, by directions and rewards or by setting a good example."

We have a moral obligation to improve parental care and support in the growth and development of youths who really need our help. (NIDA 1988).

2   The Role of Counsellors

According to the therapist Borden the client's interest and attraction towards the counsellor very much deepens the counsellor/client relationship. Having this interest creates an authentic therapeutic relationship where both the counsellor and client attract each other and are committed to work towards changes. It is important to create an atmosphere of trust, love, interest and concern to attract clients. (NIDA 1988).

As an example, John was a 17 year old male student who was a juvenile delinquent (youth crime) under probation doing community work and abiding by certain regulations. He was placed under my supervision to provide counselling and rehabilitation.

After he finished his 6 months term as a juvenile probationer, he came back and said thank you and admitted his wrongs and the kind of sufferings he had gone through. "Today I feel that I am a changed person. I realise that I have the potential to prosper and do something good to be a good person," he stated.

"One simple truth that changed me completely and why I keep coming back is that, you really understand my problems and help me a lot and I always feel the tremendous love and care you have given me. Your interest in me and my will power to change freed me from the problems I have gone through," he said.

Sometimes clients come to grief with their problems and they are moved by emotions and tear drops. Joe Mandras, who was my mentor said to me in Sogeri in 1987, "When you are lost and confused, you will shed tears, only then you will find your answers."

One of the two main components of a counselling relationship that has proven successful are the **degree of attraction** that the counsellor has for the client and the **degree of attraction** the client has for the counsellor. It is quite difficult to attract drug addicts who are living in the artificial world but if we know the art of counselling, we can handle it professionally and in an effective manner.

Effective counselling means being caring, non-judgmental, non-critical, showing love, concern and an emphatic attitude towards the clients over a period of time.

During the time of counselling, where the client is emotionally and physically disturbed and puts himself or herself in danger, we have to be more emphatic and show unconditional love and value them as persons with dignity. (NIDA 1988)

Carl Jung said, "People are living miracles and when you just listen to them emphatically, show unconditional love and reflect their feelings, healing just flows in naturally and both client and counsellor are transformed as authentic selves." We wouldn't know how and why but God is at work during human interactions. (The Addiction Letter Vol 9 1993).

The benefit of good counselling will depend on our knowledge, skills, understanding and sensitiveness of the client's problems, behaviours, attitudes, feelings, interests, concerns and personal commitments.

The counsellor's behaviour in therapeutic relationship falls under two categories. **Task (instrumental technique) and interpersonal**.

Task behaviour includes the counsellor's communications, the information provided, interventions, question providing, responses, issues raised and timing. It includes both spoken and unspoken behaviours.

Interpersonal behaviour includes the counsellor's behaviour and attitudes, manner, style and presentation of self, which also includes his or her spoken and unspoken behaviour. (NIDA 1988).

3   Confronting the Adolescents

Confrontation is seen as an intervention addressing the client's behaviours and feelings that is congruent or different or inconsistent. It is what the client is saying and what the client is experiencing in real life situations. Confrontation is done in an empathetic manner, non-judgmental, non-critical voice, without an accusatory tone but with concern.

For example: "Listen my son; you are the one who spoilt yourself in the end. You are living on alcohol and drugs which are making your life more miserable and trying to escape from problems. You may think that drinking alcohol and taking drugs gives you some good feelings but what you don't realise is it does more harm than good. You look at yourself now. You are not what you used to be in the past when you are not drinking or taking drugs."

Sometimes confrontation can result in negativity and rejection, for example: "You can't tell me that you. You are nagging me so much, just leave me alone".

Confrontation should only occur when the counsellor/client relationship is deepened with trust so that the client will not be hurt, feel threatened and leave counselling completely.

Confrontation's aim should be seen as overcoming a problem. There should be a feeling of relief when the counsellor feels close enough to counsel. This depends entirely on the client's willingness and the prevalence of a mutual relationship. The client fully accepts and is able to realise that the counsellor understands him or her realistically. (NIDA 1988).

Confrontation is an effective means to break through the psychological blockage of denial by the client. Denial of problems by youths today is very common, especially drug addicts, who are very complicated to deal with.

Drug addicts live by telling lies, taking big problem as a small issue, projecting their problems onto someone else etc.

Confrontation is an effective means to unmask denial that is part of the client's life and has been protected over a period of time. (MIDA 1988).

In confrontation, counsellors have to be fully aware of what is going to happen and to respond to it prudently. You cannot confront at will and attack in vulnerable areas that the client is trying to protect to work out a problem that has been denied. You should be interested in what he or she is not telling you.

It is important that the counsellor must know his profession and understand the term confrontation, its purpose, how to conform and the timing of the confrontation. (NIDA).

4   Clarification and Connection

To go through so many problems and human situations that threatens life, German psychologist Fritz Peris and co-founder of Gestalt therapy says patients should, **"Lose your mind and come**

to your senses."

At first the counsellor can expect to uncover only bits and pieces of the whole of the adolescent client's problems. Many of the personalities, interpersonal, psychological, physical, social and spiritual problems remain outside of the relationship. Gradually step by step we can get to all the problems. The search for the whole human person demands more than just emphatic relations to those inner reflections and changing parts. (NIDA 1988).

Gestalt therapy talks about "**the whole is more than the sum of its parts.**" The aim is to make connections between the parts and pieces of a person's whole life. Describing what the client feels or views in a given situation will not help him or her to fully know the whole problem that is affecting him or her. The adolescent will not fully understand all the implications of his or her behaviour.

The counsellor must be fully informed and must be in a position to get a holistic understanding and view of the client's problems and the possible solutions. The counsellor must assist the client to fully understand the whole picture of himself or herself and how his or her own behaviours contribute to his or her problems.

The counsellor must help the client to go beyond the point of impasse. If that cannot be achieved (being stuck) then, the impasse becomes the point of avoidance of threatening feelings, uneasiness and discomfort. (Treatment Service for Adolescence Substance, NIDA 1988).

In order to help the client, the counsellor has to be fully in touch with them and they must also comply with the counsellor. Gestalt therapy maintains that an authentic therapeutic relationship between the counsellor and the client will entail changes in both parties. (Refer gestalt therapy in the following paragraphs).

5 Self-Disclosure

In human relations in order to dig deep and explore another person's life and behaviour we have to reveal our personalities. It may happen that a repressed, suppressed and hidden psychological conflict in an adolescent will not be revealed until the counsellor is able to express his or her own feelings.

There are risks involved and we have to be careful in our newly formed relationship, even though it can be a new and healthy experience. Experienced counsellors are able to guard themselves against risks while being fully aware of filling spaces with personal elements and are alert and open to creating insights and unique experiences. (NIDA 1988).

Self-disclosure is only allowed when the counsellor shares his or her experiences with the client to benefit the client. It must be clear, meaningful and relevant to the client's problems and situations.

Self-disclosure is used with an accurate sense of timing and in a manner appropriate for the client to make use of it. It is never used for the counsellor's own needs.

The clear and non-judgmental disclosure of how the counsellor is affected by the client's feelings and thoughts and his or her responses and actions place the client in a better position to understand his or her own difficulties in life. The counsellor self-discloses his or her reactions to the client's experiences and situations. (NIDA 1988).

Chapter 17

Gestalt Therapy

FRITZ PERLS, a Jewish psychologist and one of the co-founders of gestalt therapy mentioned that it is something that is rediscovered and explored within ourselves and inherited in nature.

Even though he was a genius he humbled himself by saying that he did not invent anything special and that it was not something new, rather it was something borrowed from other concepts.

Gestalt therapy tries to rediscover the inner psychological and spiritual energy that is already inbuilt within the self and which needs to be fully utilised and explored rather than looking externally to gain support. (The Addiction Letter Vol. 9, 1993).

Gestalt therapy looks beyond the impulse and tries to work on the blockages that stop progressive growth.

The point beyond impulse is something that is a threat because at most times we really don't want to talk about ourselves or want other people to know our secrets and faults and we pretend that we don't have a problem. We normally put a mask on as protective armour and don't reveal our personalities but that is threatening to our genuine self. Gestalt therapy helps us explore beyond our impulses and tries to free us of this life threatening blockage. (The Addiction Letter Vol. 9, 1993).

Gestalt therapy sees the whole as greater than the sum of its parts. We are made of the bits and pieces of a whole human person but the sum of that whole human person is much greater than the single bits and pieces. (The Addiction Letter, Vol. 9, 1993).

According to Bill Schetz, a gestalt therapist, there are six levels or dimensions which make up the whole human person and they are **spiritual, physical, social, psychological, interpersonal and emotional**. All these dimensions makes up the human person as a wholly authentic and unique being.

In gestalt therapy counsellor and client develop a therapeutic and authentic relationship. Exploring this relationship holistically entails both the counsellor and the client changing and growing. (The Addiction Letter, Vol. 9, 1993).

One of gestalt therapy's major foundations is the belief that all of our coping mechanisms are creative adjustments towards the stresses of life and depend on the makeup of the individual's personality. They are creative because they are chosen among several alternatives and because they alter our experience in some way. (The Addiction Letter, Vol. 9, 1993).

Bill Schetz explained the gestalt therapy notion with an illustration of a box of wooden blocks.

Suppose we have a box containing 12 blocks, do we see any special feature? No.

If we take the blocks out and align (organize) them so that they are in a configuration of an orderly manner or pattern, then we can see a single figure. The 12 blocks become a unified totality; an organised meaningful whole. (NAADAC, Newsletter, Vol. 1, 1995).

When we apply this example to human beings we will discover that all the bits and pieces of a human life becomes something more and greater as a unified holistic person.

Gestalt therapy works towards achieving holistic or authentic human growth by encouraging, supporting and completing unfinished business and assisting the clients towards their own inbuilt potential, self-actualization, internal beauty, love, wisdom, knowledge and capacity for growth. (NAADAC, Newsletter, Vol. 1, 1995).

The gestalt therapy awareness or experience and contact cycle can be summed up as follows;

When healthy persons are thirsty their need for water becomes apparent:

➢ Through the awareness of sensation (dry throat).
➢ Through identification of need (I am thirsty).
➢ Through the activation of energy (go to the water tap).
➢ To action (pouring water and drinking it).
➢ To contact (cool water – feels good).
➢ To enjoy the need-satisfaction and withdrawal, leading to organismic homeostasis (no longer thirsty).

When this natural completion of the cycle becomes blocked, dysfunctional behaviours appears and individuals have problems in their behaviour patterns. Drug addicts and alcoholics need alcohol and drugs and cannot emerge as whole people. The awareness contact withdrawal cycle is interrupted through misidentification of sensations and inappropriate need fulfilment. Eventually behaviours become rigid, and then they become addictive patterns that do not allow self-regulation and homeostasis to occur. (Addiction Letter, Vol. 9, 1993).

Examining the Interruptions

In addiction recovery, it is important that this life cycle and its interruptions be examined in the context of the individual's problems, relationships and its social and environmental aspects.

The gestalt ten step recovery programs for addiction recovery organises the evaluation of the client's life style in the context of awareness. This makes individuals feel responsible for their own problems; life stresses decisions and choices, relations and their holistic life. (Addiction Letter, Vol. 9, 1993).

Chapter 18

Ten Steps to Addiction Recovery

THE ten steps toward addiction recovery are:

1. When I drink and take drugs I suffer too much and make my life unmanageable.

2. I am aware that I have choices. By utilizing choices fully, I can create a less troubled life.

3. I am capable of discovering enriching support within myself and in relation to others.

4. I understand that my difficulties and successes were created in relationship with others and in the context of my environment. I can courageously examine my own and others' contribution to them.

5. I am willing to work on this unfinished business because it interferes with the fulfilments of my hopes and I accept that joy and pain are part of the human condition.

6. I have the strength to live life in the present and become strengthened through giving and receiving relationships.

7. I am aware that I have freedoms and responsibilities towards myself and others and will meet them with concern for those involved.

8. I accept myself as fully human and capable of any human deed. With respect to the integrity of each person, I will strive to enrich myself and others.

9. I am interested in differences in attitudes, values and perceptions and welcome them if I can use them to improve understanding of others.

10. I express my spirit in the deeds and my personal relations. (Helga M Matzko, 1993).

The first three steps stress personal decisions and choice processes by examining others people's contributions to problems and works towards an examination of life style and the rediscovery of long abandoned internal and external support. Steps four and five allow us to examine our problem development as part of a process in connection with others at particular time and place. In addition, it stresses that we should examine the coping skills that helps us to survive.

Chapter 19

What are the Steps in Drug Awareness?

AWARENESS education means to make people aware and know that there is a drug problem; enough to destroy life. Let them understand the seriousness of the problems. Let them feel the pain and from feeling the effects of drugs and pain they will find their own solutions.

Awareness education of the general population should aim at:

A. Demand Reduction

Demand reduction means to reduce the consumption rate and it aims at educating people on the effects of alcohol and drug abuse and its dire consequences. We should talk about the human lives that are affected by drugs. We should also talk about why people are taking drugs and the behaviours associated with drugs and the consequences.

B. Supply Reduction

Supply reduction means our awareness should aim at the legal implications: what the law says and the penalties for cultivating drugs, selling and trafficking them, home brew production and marketing and also the physical, social, psychological, spiritual, moral and environmental effects.

Demand and supply reduction both have separate roles to play and in order to solve the drug problem we need to address both together.

People come in contact with drugs and alcohol because they are readily available for consumption or use.

People want to experiment out of curiosity and try to find out what is all about. People in PNG are great believers in magic and it could be a magic drink or plant to find secrets.

People take alcohol and drugs as a coping behaviour to control tensions, problems and life pressures.

People take drugs and alcohol because their bodies wants it. They have already developed tolerance and dependency. They are addicted drinkers or drug addicts.

C. <u>Our Target Population</u>

➢ Those who are consumers of narcotic drugs, home brew and other illegal drugs.

➢ Our target population should also involve the drug cultivators, traffickers and home brew producers and sellers.

➢ Those who can influence other people against taking drugs, for example, church workers, community leaders, youth leaders, women leaders, peace mediators, magistrates, teachers, health workers, social workers, police, CIS and so on.

➢ Those who are at the high risk of taking drugs, especially youths and adolescences who are at the cross roads between childhood and complicated adult life.

D. Our Approach to Different Target Groups

In our approach to school children, we should talk about preventive measures. Do not take drugs, it will spoil your body, your mind and spirit. Taking drugs spoils your education and there is no hope for your future. Primary school children must be educated separately from high school and tertiary students.

The village youths and other adults must be educated separately. The more people are educated and informed on the dangers of drugs and alcohol abuse, the more they will understand the side effects.

Awareness can be carried out with more information on the dangers of drugs, the physical effects, psychological effects, social effects and law and order problems. They must be made aware of what is going on. People must be made aware and learn to look at themselves, their families and the community they live in and what drug abuse is doing to them and society in general.

People have to be stimulated to know these problems are spoiling their wellbeing and they themselves have to find workable solutions. Empowering people to recognise drug problems and to find their own solutions is an effective means. People should take ownership of drug problems and address their own problems, rather than turning to other people to solve them for them.

E. Things Required for Educational Awareness

1. To be fully informed on the topic of drugs and alcohol abuse.
2. Awareness aids and materials.
3. Posters on alcohol and drug abuse and other related topics

like child abuse.

4. Booklets.

5. A loud hailer or PA system.

F. <u>How to Draw Audiences</u>

Awareness goes well with drama, songs, outreach programs, bible sharing and other activities in church. Awareness in church networking works effectively and people get the message in this sort of spiritually rich and sober environment.

G. The Response from the Audience

> Allow time for questions and comments from the audience.

> Expect some criticisms and outbursts of temper from some people, especially those who support drug habits.

> Do not allow other people to add on what you have said. He or she might give false information and confuse the people.

> Allow commentators who are supportive of your awareness and suggest plans of action.

> Answer the questions that you know the answer to or are capable of answering but do not make any attempt to answer questions that you don't know the answer to. You can refer the person to someone who can answer his or her questions.

Chapter 20

Human Rights

(The rights of the drug addicts).

ALL human beings, including alcoholics and drug addicts, have certain rights as well as obligations. Since World War 11 a lot of emphasis been given to the rights of human beings because wars have no respect and values for human beings. Even during normal times in our contemporary world we see a lot of violation of human rights.

These rights have been described by the United Nations in a declaration entitled the Universal Declaration of Human Rights, issued on 10th December, 1948.

This first declarations of human rights were politically oriented but since then many more "declarations" have been written and agreed upon by the member states of the UN, for example, the Rights for the Child.

The Declaration of Human Rights is based on the recognition of the human dignity we have. This human dignity or value is explained by people in different ways based on religious beliefs, tradition and ethics.

Christians base human dignity on the belief of creation from God and their special relationship with Him as child and father.

The Christians' basis comes from the very beginning of the Bible where in Genesis it states that God created man in his own image and likeness. This image and likeness provides us with an immortal life, a life that lives forever and that has an eternal destiny with God.

The Universal Declaration of Human Rights states in Article 3 that "Everyone has a right to life, liberty and security of person". Article 4 prohibits slavery and ensures that everyone has the right to be free from slavery.

These human rights include the right to be happy, to enjoy life and to be free from fear.

Anyone who has had anything to do with drug abuse knows very well how much drugs have taken away rights to life, liberty and happiness. The right to life cannot be limited only to the rights not to be murdered or killed unjustly. Drugs kill not only the user but also others through drug related crimes.

Those who push drugs, the traffickers and the suppliers, are contributing to the unjust killing, often of youths who are vulnerable to drug taking.

Just as a prisoner can be held behind bars a drug user is chained by his or her habits and misery.

Article 1 says, "All human beings are born free and equal in dignity and rights; they are endowed with reason and conscience and should act towards one another in the spirit of brotherhood."

Nothing could be further from acting towards "one another in a spirit of brotherhood" than drug abuse.

As is clearly seen the drug abuser harms not only himself but also his fellow human beings and that is certainly not acting in "the spirit of brotherhood."

Nor does the drug trafficker and supplier act in the spirit of brotherhood when he poisons the life and minds of those who take up drugs to make it through life.

It is also difficult to understand how some governments in the world can appear to support the United Nations and at the same time be corrupt in allowing drug trafficking to go on in their country.

It is difficult to understand how some persons can advocate the legalizing of drugs like marijuana when there is an abundance of information and research on what drug abuse is doing to individuals and society.

Chapter 21

A Guide for Parents, Teachers & Guardians

Signs and Symptoms of Drug Abuse

THE following may be signs of drug abuse. However, they can also be signs of other illness or general health.

➢ Reddened or watery eyes.
➢ Dilated or pin-pointed pupils.
➢ Sudden loss of weight.
➢ Occasional memory loss.
➢ Slurred and slow speech.
➢ Lack of energy.
➢ Disturbed sleep patterns.
➢ Chronic coughing.
➢ Poor coordination (staggering or stumbling movements).
➢ Loss of appetite but a craving for sweets - called the "munchies".

The following signs are not proof of drug abuse but they may be indicators. Some of these signs can simply be a part of growing up.

➢ Loss of enthusiasm and involvement.
➢ Withdrawal from hobbies and sports.
➢ Reluctance to introduce new friends.
➢ Staying away from home or school without explanation.
➢ Initiating and/or over reacting to criticism.
➢ Loss of interest and deterioration in the quality of school

work.
➢ Unusual requests for money.
➢ Sudden changes in mood and behaviour.
➢ Lack of pride in personal appearance.
➢ Frequent unexplained phone calls.
➢ Loss of concentration.
➢ Cigarette rolling papers.
➢ Collecting small spoons.
➢ Collecting empty bottles and beer cans.

How to Assist in the Children's Problems

➢ Don't panic or over-react.
➢ Try to find out all you can without showing too much anxiety.
➢ Establish the facts and stick to them.
➢ Discuss the facts with your son or daughter.
➢ Don't moralize or preach.
➢ Support your son or daughter by showing understanding and concern.
➢ Identifying positive ways of correcting the situation.
➢ Make them responsible for their own drug use.

Chapter 22

Summary

BRIEFLY, although each person as an individual has the right and free will to decide whether to take drugs or not, one must not abuse that right. All must bear in mind that there is only one life and that no person is an island, meaning that all people co-exist and everyone has a responsibility to make sure that the exercising of one's rights and freedoms does not become an impediment or danger to the rights, wellbeing and healthy existence of those around them.

As we have discussed in the book, most drugs are dangerous and can cause severe psychological or physiological damage to the user.

Drug use can also have consequences on one's family, community and society through the actions of the addicts when they are under the influence of drugs.

And the social costs, such as rehabilitation and counselling, medication, legal and correctional services etc. can be huge, affecting other development programs and endeavours.

Hence next time you feel the urge to take a drug, you must think twice about the effects and consequences of that action upon yourself, the community and society at large.

The good values of responsibility, discipline, sacrifice, wise thinking, choice making and the basic rights of freedom rests within each and every individual.

The best thing all of us can do is say no to any form of drug that is classified as illicit because it is dangerous and destructive to our body, mind and those around us.

If we have already become hooked, and as long as we are alive, it is not too late to seek help, both mental counselling and rehabilitation and, physical medication.

All people have the inner ability and willpower to free themselves from the bondage of drugs and alcoholism. All one has to do is to take a bold step forward and say no to drugs and at the same time seek appropriate help and your life can change for the better.

You are born to be free from bondage, including drugs and alcohol. You can be free.

Glossary

1. **Abstinence** – not partaking of/in an activity such as drinking or drug taking.

2. **Addiction** – the condition where an alcoholic or the drug addict develops physiological and psychological dependence upon a chemical substance and has already developed tolerance to it.

3. **Addictive** – when two drugs acting similarly are taken at the same time and the result is greater.

4. **Supra-addictive** – when the effects of two synergistic drugs are greater than the sum of their individual potency.

5. **Alcohol** – (ethanol) is a general anaesthetic. It depresses the Central Nervous System and affects other bodily functions.

6. **Amphetamine Type Stimulants (ATS)** - name of a synthetic drug or designer drug produced in underground laboratories.

7. **Antiretroviral drugs** – they are manufactured licit drugs of recent nature. When antiretroviral drugs are given to people living with HIV AIDS it replicates immune responses and healthy living conditions improves.

8. **Analgesic** – a pain reliever that does not make a person unconscious.

9. **Anorexia Nervosa** – an eating disorder characterised by

psychological disorder and distorted bodily image.

10. **Antagonism** – the action of one drug will eliminate the effects of the other, e.g. Valium will counteract the sleeplessness caused by stimulants.

11. **Barbiturates** – classes of drugs derived from barbituric acid that act as depressants to the central nervous system (CNS).

12. **Biological** – relating to or produced by biological process.

13. **Behaviour** – defined as observable or measurable movement of an organism.

14. **Cannabis** – scientific name for marijuana plant, either *Cannabis sativa, Cannabis indica* or *Cannabis ruderalis*.

15. **Cardiovascular** – the blood circulatory system and includes heart, veins and arteries.

16. **Cerebral** – relating to the brain or the intellect.

17. **Chasing the dragon** – a popular Chinese expression describing inhaling of drugs.

18. **Chemical Dependency** – when one takes in drugs which are not a normal bodily need that the body has to cope and convert into the normal functions of the body. Chemical dependency means you are dependent on a drug that your body had already got used to it and you can't get rid of it e.g. when you don't have smoke you don't do anything else until you find a cigarette.

19. **Cirrhosis** – referring to a liver problem caused by excessive use of alcohol which develops scar tissues in the liver,

which does not function normally and is a major cause of deaths among alcoholics.

20. **Cognitive** – related to brain function, reasoning and perception.

21. **Code of ethics** – principles or guiding rules governing an individual or group.

22. **Compulsive behaviour** – acting abnormal due to heavy drinking that does not make any sense to others.

23. **Cross tolerance** – a person who has developed tolerance to one drug will show the same effect to another drug. For example, alcoholics taking in sedatives or stimulants or anaesthetics or other similar drugs without effect because of the tolerance to the central nervous system already created by the alcohol.

24. **Delirium** – a mental disorder which has resulted in confusion, disorientation, experience of hallucinations, delusions and depression.

25. **Delirium Tremens** – extreme mental disturbances or psychological problems with tremors that is caused by excessive and prolonged alcohol and drug use.

26. **Delusions** – feeling of having super human powers reinforced by imaginations.

27. **Deviant behaviour** – someone behaving outside of the normal ethical standards of behaviour in a given society.

28. **Deviance** – is a characteristics of a criminal behaviour that has conflicts with society.

29. **Drug** – any substance that, when taken into the human body, may modify one of more of its functions.

30. **Drug substitution therapy** – prescribed drug medication given to drug dependency patients under strict medical supervision to eliminate or replace the dependency producing substances.

31. **Dysfunctional** – describing a behaviour process which adversely affects individuals and families.

32. **Ethanol** – a particular form of alcohol with the chemical component of C_2H_60.

33. **Ethyl alcohol** – is alcohol that is fermented or distilled that is a volatile, flammable liquid with intoxicating properties.

34. **Etiology** – the study of origin and causes of diseases.

35. **Euphoria** – the false hope of feeling good with no problems at all.

36. **Genetic** – referring to genetics, pertaining to genes.

37. **Habituation** – refers to the alcoholics or the drug addicts' attitude that the effects produced by the chemical or the situation associated with its use, are necessary to maintain well-being, can become a craving or compulsion.

38. **Hallucinogen** - a drug that induces perceptions of things, seeing things, hearing of voices and feeling things that do not exist.

39. **Hallucination** – three types:

    a.   **Auditory hallucination** – Hearing voices and noises

that are not there.

b. **Visual hallucination** - seeing things and objects that are not there.

c. **Tactile hallucination** – feeling things on your body that are not there.

40. **Harm reduction** – working towards reducing severe physical, psychological, social, legal, moral and medical problems associated with drugs with effective intervention and preventive measures.

41. **Hyper** –increasing, larger, bigger or above normal.

42. **Hypertension** – relating to high blood pressure.

43. **Illegal** - against the law.

44. **Intoxication** - The state of getting drunk due to alcohol consumption which results in slurred speech, impaired motor coordination, impaired sensory perceptions and impaired moral judgment.

45. **Korsakov syndrome** – referring to brain damage after excessive use of alcohol.

46. **Moral** – the principle of right or wrong, good or bad value or dis-value in behaviour. Ethics also express morality and its principles.

47. **Moral inventory** – making a stock take of wrong or right, good or bad, accepted or unaccepted behaviour one has committed and defects of character.

48. **Morphine** – is a sedative drug derived from the opium

poppy plant.

49. **Mortality** – relating to death.

50. **Narcotic** – an opiate or natural or synthetic opium derivative that in moderate doses dulls the senses and relieves pain and induces consumers to sleep.

51. **Natural** – drugs which occur in nature or are isolated and refined from naturally occurring substances.

52. **Nature** – heredity or inherited traits.

53. **Nurture** - physical or social environment

54. **Neurotransmitters** – chemical messages in the brain system.

55. **Pathological** – based on a disease, not normal or healthy.

56. **Pathology** – a structural or functional imbalance in the family, rather than hardships being faced by any single individual within the family.

57. **Pharmacological** – relating to or determined by pharmacology.

58. **Pharmacology** – The properties of reaction to drugs.

59. **Physiological Dependence** – a physical condition where an alcoholic or a drug addicts' physical or bodily system has made a cellular adaption to the continuous consumption of drugs and when discontinued will suffer withdrawal symptoms.

60. **Psychological dependence** – a mental condition where an alcoholic or a drug addicts' thinking process and behaviour

is already converted to consume more drugs and when stopped will experience withdrawal symptoms.

61. **Poly drug abuse** – The habit of taking two or more drugs at the same time.

62. **Relapse** – relapse is defined as a progressive pattern of behaviour which permits symptoms of disease to become reactivated in a person who had previously suffered those symptoms.

63. **Sincemilla** – name of hybrid cannabis which is seedless.

64. **Sociological** – the study of sociology directed towards needs and problems.

65. **Spirituality** – our relationship with our higher power with prayer and meditation.

66. **Synergism** – synergism means the effects of two or more drugs taken together that add more effects or double the effects of each individual drug added together. That means the joint effects of alcohol and cannabis or any other drug is greater than the original effects or may produce severe side effects.

67. **Tetrahydrocanabinol (THC)** – the main cannabinoids (chemical component) or drug in cannabis plant.

68. **Tolerance** – The body gets used to the drug so one has to take in more and more doses to feel the same effects.

69. **Toxicity** – poisonous, or dangerous drugs.

70. **Transactional Analysis** – when people interact as parent,

adult and child.

71. **Withdrawal** – means reducing the intake of drugs or stopping the use of drugs.

72. **Withdrawal symptoms** – is the sickness or symptoms caused by not taking drugs which have become part of the normal physical/psychological functioning e.g. one gets head-aches and feel sick when he doesn't drink alcohol.

Bibliography

Shirley Trickett
Coming Off Tranquilizers & Sleeping Pills
1991

UN Office on Drugs and Crime
Update November 2003.

Steven E Gardner, DSW
Drug and Alcohol Abuse
Implications for Treatment
National Institute on Drug Abuse
5600 Fishers Lane
Rockville, Maryland
1987

Eric Berne
Games People Play
Psychology of Human Relationships
Penguin Books Limited
Great Britain 1964

CEIDA
PMB No 6 P.O ROZELLE
NSW 2039
Australia 1991

Nancy Chodorow

Psychoanalysis and the Sociology of Gender
University of California Press 1978

Henry Peschke
Christian Ethics
Alcester and Dublin 1979

ACCORD Report
Bali, Indonesia November 2001.

National Institute on Drug Abuse
Treatment Research Monograph Serious
Rockville, Maryland 20857
USA 1989

Thomas Borkman
National Institute on Alcohol Abuse and Alcoholism
Rockville, Maryland USA

An Initiative of the Simbu Writer's Association

www.ingramcontent.com/pod-product-compliance
Lightning Source LLC
Chambersburg PA
CBHW072026190526
45166CB00015B/510